A Pocket Obstetric

A Pocket Obstetrics and Gynaecology

Sir Stanley G. Clayton
MD MS (Lond.) FRCP FRCS FRCOG
Late Emeritus Professor of Obstetrics and
Gynaecology, King's College Hospital Medical
School, University of London. Honorary
Consulting Obstetric and Gynaecological
Surgeon, Queen Charlotte's Hospital and
Chelsea Hospital for Women, London.

John R. Newton
MD BS (Lond.) FRCOG
Lawson Tait Professor of Obstetrics and
Gynaecology, University of Birmingham.

ELEVENTH EDITION

CHURCHILL LIVINGSTONE
EDINBURGH LONDON AND NEW YORK 1988

CHURCHILL LIVINGSTONE
Medical Division of Longman Group UK Limited

Distributed in the United States of America by Churchill
Livingstone Inc., 1560 Broadway, New York, N.Y. 10036, and
by associated companies, branches and representatives throughout
the world.

Copyright J. & A. Churchill Limited 1948
© Longman Group Limited 1979
© Longman Group UK Limited 1988

All rights reserved. No part of this publication may be
reproduced, stored in a retrieval system, or transmitted in any
form or by any means, electronic, mechanical, photocopying,
recording or otherwise, without the prior permission of the
publishers (Churchill Livingstone, Robert Stevenson House, 1–3
Baxter's Place, Leith Walk, Edinburgh, EH1 3AF).

First Edition 1948	Sixth Edition 1967
Second Edition 1952	Seventh Edition 1972
Third Edition 1956	Eighth Edition 1976
Fourth Edition 1961	Ninth Edition 1979
Fifth Edition 1965	Tenth Edition 1983
	Eleventh Edition 1988

ISBN 0-443-03777-9

British Library Cataloguing in Publication Data
Clayton, Stanley G.
 A pocket obstetrics and gynaecology. — 11th ed.
 1. Gynecology 2. Obstetrics
 I. Title II. Newton, John R. III. Clayton, Stanley G.
Pocket obstetrics 618   RG101

Library of Congress Cataloging in Publication Data
Clayton, Stanley George, Sir.
 A pocket obstetrics and gynaecology.
 Rev. ed. of: A pocket obstetrics. 10th ed. 1983.
 Includes index.
 1. Obstetrics — Handbooks, manuals, etc. I. Newton, John
R. (John Richard) II. Clayton, Stanley George, Sir. A pocket
Obstetrics. III. Title. [DNLM:
1. Gynecology — handbooks. 2. Obstetrics — handbooks.
WQ 39 C625p]
RG531.C48 1987   618.2   87-760

Produced by Longman Singapore Publishers (Pte) Ltd.
Printed in Singapore.

Preface

In this pocket book we have tried to present the basic information about obstetrics and gynaecology that an undergraduate student may need.

The book was first published in 1948, and has hitherto been in two volumes. The present eleventh edition is in a single volume, and this will allow better integration of descriptions of normal function, obstetric abnormalities and gynaecological disorders, with some further economy of words.

For doctors facts are essential, but in treating a woman's problems and anxieties understanding is also required, which can only be gained by talking to patients and watching their progress in the clinics, wards and theatres, where we hope this small book will be a useful companion.

S. G. C.
1988 J. R. N.

APPRECIATION

Sadly, Sir Stanley Clayton died after undertaking the revision and rewriting of this, the first joint publication of *A Pocket Obstetrics* and *A Pocket Gynaecology*, both in their eleventh editions. It is hoped that this book will continue to provide students and doctors with a useful companion, while, at the same time, providing a small memorial to an influential exponent of these sciences.

Contents

A. NORMAL FUNCTION

1. **The menstrual cycle and ovulation** — 3
2. **Normal pregnancy** — 16
   Fertilization and embedding of the ovum. Physiology of pregnancy. Symptoms and signs. Diagnosis. Antenatal care.
3. **Normal labour** — 34
   Stages. The bony pelvis. Pelvic floor. Fetal measurements. Mechanism of labour. Management of normal labour.
4. **Normal puerperium** — 56
   Physiology. Management. Postnatal care.

B. OBSTETRIC ABNORMALITIES

5. **Abnormal pregnancy** — 63
   Abortion. Hydatidiform mole. Choriocarcinoma. Ectopic pregnancy. Vomiting. Hypertension and proteinuria. Pyelonephritis. Polyhydramnios. Placental pathology. Antepartum haemorrhage. Preterm labour. Premature rupture of membranes. Postmaturity. Intrauterine fetal death. Pelvic tumours and uterine abnormalities complicating pregnancy. General disorders complicating pregnancy. Drugs and the fetus.
6. **Abnormal labour** — 115
   Delay in labour. Malpresentations. Fetal malformations. Disproportion. Abnormal uterine action. Obstructed labour. Multiple pregnancy. Prolapse of the cord. Postpartum haemorrhage. Retention of the placenta. Coagulation disorders. Obstetrical injuries. Shock.

7. Abnormal puerperium — 154
Puerperal pyrexia. Abnormalities of the breast. Venous thrombosis. Pituitary necrosis. Renal necrosis. Mental illness.

8. The fetus at risk in late pregnancy and during labour — 166

9. Haemolytic disease — 168

10. Obstetric operations — 173
Induction of labour. Forceps. Vacuum extraction. Pudendal block. Epidural analgesia. Caesarean section. Amniocentesis. Oxytocic drugs.

11. Care of the newborn child — 189
Asphyxia neonatorum. Other immediate care. Breast feeding. Artificial feeding. Small infants. Birth injuries. Other abnormalities.

12. Obstetric statistics — 208

C. GYNAECOLOGICAL DISORDERS

13. Gynaecological investigation — 215

14. Embryology and congenital abnormalities — 217

15. Pelvic injuries and displacements — 228
Injuries. Anatomy of pelvic supports. Prolapse. Retroversion. Inversion.

16. Infective diseases — 236
Sexually transmitted diseases. Vulvitis. Vaginitis. Cervicitis and endometritis. Salpingo-oöphoritis. Pelvic peritonitis and cellulitis. Tuberculosis.

17. Tumours — 260
Vulval, urethral and vaginal tumours. Uterine tumours. Ovarian tumours. Tumours of broad ligament and tube. Endometriosis.

18. Functional disorders of menstruation — 302
Amenorrhoea. Anovular menstruation. Dysfunctional bleeding. Dysmenorrhoea.

19. Menopausal symptoms — 316

20. Dyspareunia — 319

21. Infertility — 320

22. Endocrine preparations — 329

23. Contraception, sterilization and termination of pregnancy	334
24. Backache in women	350
25. Urinary disorders in gynaecological patients	351
26. Notes on gynaecological operations	357
Index	370

SECTION A

Normal function

1

The menstrual cycle and ovulation

The activity of the whole female reproductive system is directed by the hypothalamus, whose *gonadotrophic releasing hormone* (GnRH) controls the secretion of gonadotrophic hormones from the anterior pituitary gland. There are two gonadotrophic hormones, *follicle stimulating hormone* (FSH) and *luteinizing hormone* (LH). In response to the gonadotrophins the ripening ovarian follicle secretes *oestradiol*, and after ovulation the corpus luteum secretes both *oestradiol and progesterone*. These hormones act on the uterus and other reproductive organs; they also control the release of hormones from the hypothalamus and pituitary by a feedback mechanism (p. 11).

During pregnancy hormones are also secreted by the placenta (p. 17).

The hypothalamus

The hypothalamus is a small band of grey matter situated directly above the pituitary gland. It secretes GnRH in pulses into the hypophyseal venous plexus in the pituitary stalk, by which the GnRH is conveyed to specific hormone-producing cells in the anterior pituitary. GnRH is sometimes referred to as luteinizing hormone releasing hormone (LHRH) but, as it also releases FSH, gonadotrophic releasing hormone is a more correct description. It is a decapeptide.

The anterior pituitary gland

The pituitary gland weighs about 0.5 g and consists of two lobes. The anterior lobe contains several types of secretory cells. Immunological studies have shown that the basophil cells (gonadotrophs) secrete FSH and LH, whereas the acidophil cells secrete *prolactin*, a hormone concerned with normal lactation.

LH and FSH are released in pulses by hypothalamic releasing hormone, but prolactin secretion is held in check by a hypothalamic inhibiting factor. If hypothalamic function fails FSH and LH levels fall and prolactin levels rise.

FSH and LH are both glycoproteins which are excreted in the urine, and can be estimated there and in the blood by radioimmunoassay.

The ovaries

Ovarian (Graafian) follicles are seen in the ovaries in various stages of ripeness. The primitive follicle consists of a central large cell, the oöcyte, surrounded by a single ring of cells. As the follicle ripens the cells around the oöcyte proliferate to become several layers deep, and are known as granulosa cells. As the granulosa cells increase in number, a displacing fluid appears, and splits them into a smaller mass of cells surrounding the oöcyte (cumulus oöphorus) and a larger sheet of cells that line the follicle. Outside the granulosa cells is a layer of smaller theca-interna cells, and outside these the ovarian stroma is condensed to form the theca externa (Fig. 1.1). The oöcyte is about 0.1 mm in diameter with an eccentric nucleus and nucleolus. The ripe follicle is about 20 mm in diameter and its size can be observed by ultrasonic examination.

At birth the ovary contains thousands of follicles, but only one ripens fully in each normal menstrual cycle. This follicle

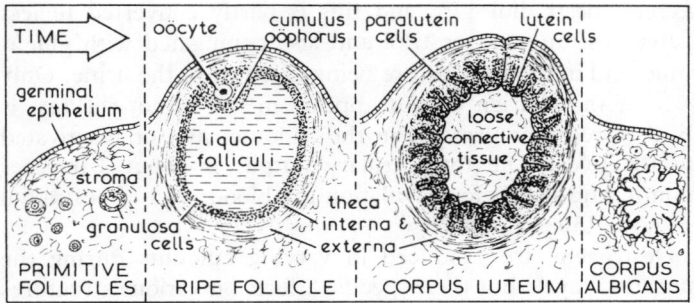

Fig. 1.1 Diagram of Graafian follicle and corpus luteum.

approaches the surface of the ovary as it enlarges, and at ovulation the oöcyte and a few surrounding granulosa cells are discharged into the peritoneal cavity. After ovulation the follicle becomes the *corpus luteum*. The granulosa cells lining the follicle accumulate lipoid and are now called lutein cells, and a similar change occurs in the theca-interna cells, which are now called paralutein cells. Both layers become infolded into the cavity of the follicle. When the corpus luteum finally degenerates it shrinks into a hyaline mass, the *corpus albicans*.

The ovarian hormones

The ovary is stimulated by gonadotrophins to produce steroid hormones. Oestrogens are primarily responsible for the development and maintenance of the sex organs and the secondary sexual characteristics, and for the menstrual cycle, while progesterone has an additive effect, being necessary for the secretory response of the endometrium and implantation of the ovum.

Oestrogens

There are several oestrogenic steroids. The ovary chiefly

secretes oestradiol 17β, and this is partly converted to less active oestrone and oestriol and also conjugated with glucuronic acid in the liver before being excreted in the urine. Only 10% of the ovarian output appears in the urine; the rest is fixed to receptor proteins in the endometrium or inactivated by the liver. The total urinary output is about 1 mg per month, and just before ovulation the blood level of oestradiol is above 1500 pmol/l.

Oestrogens are produced in varying amounts during the menstrual cycle but their specific effects on various structures may be listed:

Vulva: vascularity and enlargement of labia.
Vagina: epithelial proliferation, with cornification and accumulation of glycogen in cells.
Cervix: secretion of clear mucus at the time of ovulation. If this midcycle mucus is allowed to dry on a microscope slide a fern-like pattern of salt crystals forms.
Uterine and tubal muscle: hypertrophy and increased contractility.
Endometrium: increased vascularity and proliferation of both glands and stroma. Oestrogens acting intermittently, as in menstrual cycles, produce normal proliferation, but if oestrogens act continuously for several weeks pathological hyperplasia occurs.
Breasts: duct proliferation.
Secondary sexual characteristics: growth of pubic and axillary hair, feminine fat distribution, feminine psyche.

Oestrogens also have negative feedback effects on the hypothalamus (p. 11).

The chemistry of ovarian steroids and synthetic oestrogens is described on p. 331.

Progesterone

Progesterone is the principal steroid produced by the corpus luteum in the second half of the menstrual cycle, when the daily production rate is 25 mg; at other times it is less than 5 mg, but there is a low but constant level of progesterone in the blood because it is produced by the adrenal cortex as well as the ovary. After ovulation the blood level of progesterone is at least 30 nmol/l. About 20% of the progesterone is excreted in the urine as pregnanediol glucuronide, which can be estimated chemically.

Following the action of oestrogens the specific effects of progesterone on various organs are:

Vagina: the epithelial cells become more basophilic and clump together in a smear.
Cervical mucus: after ovulation a smaller amount of viscid mucus is formed, which does not show ferning on drying.
Endometrium: secretory change and decidual reaction occur (p. 9).
Uterine and tubal muscle: stronger, though slower, contractions occur.
Breasts: if duct proliferation has been induced by oestrogens proliferation of acini follows.
Body temperature: at the time of ovulation the basal temperature rises 0.5°C, and this elevation is maintained until the next period.

The chemistry of progesterone and of synthetic progestogens is described on p. 333.

Androgens

Androgens are metabolic precursors of oestrogens, and are produced by the ovary, especially by the stromal cells, and also by the adrenal cortex. The principal ovarian androgens are androstenedione and dehydroepiandrosterone (DHA). Androgens help to maintain female libido.

The menstrual cycle

For convenience of description the normal adult function is described before the changes which occur at puberty. The normal menstrual cycle lasts 28 days, including 5 days of bleeding. The first day of the period is conventionally taken to be the first day of the cycle. No woman is absolutely regular, and cycles of 25 to 32 days can be accepted as normal.

From the 5th day of the cycle the ripening follicle secretes oestrogen and the blood level rises steadily until shortly before ovulation, which takes place at about the 14th day. After ovulation there is a fall in the oestrogen level, and then a smaller secondary rise (Figs. 1.2 and 1.3). During the second half of the cycle the corpus luteum secretes both oestrogen and progesterone, and the blood level of both hormones reaches a peak 6 to 7 days before menstruation is due. If the oöcyte liberated in that cycle is not fertilized there is a fall in the level of both hormones, and menstruation occurs.

Immediately after menstruation the uterus is lined by a simple cubical epithelium, with short tubular glands and scanty interglandular stroma. Under the influence of oestrogens the endometrium becomes more vascular, and the tubular glands longer, with columnar cells (*proliferative phase*). After ovulation, when the action of progesterone is added, the glands secrete mucus, so that each gland is distended and has a crenated outline. The stromal cells swell and are now called decidual cells, and the stroma becomes more compact, especially near the surface (*secretory phase*). If a fertilized ovum embeds in the endometrium this decidual reaction persists, otherwise menstruation occurs and the endometrium breaks down. This disintegration is due to ischaemic necrosis, as the endometrial arterioles contract and cut off the blood supply to all but the deepest layer. Endo-

THE MENSTRUAL CYCLE AND OVULATION 9

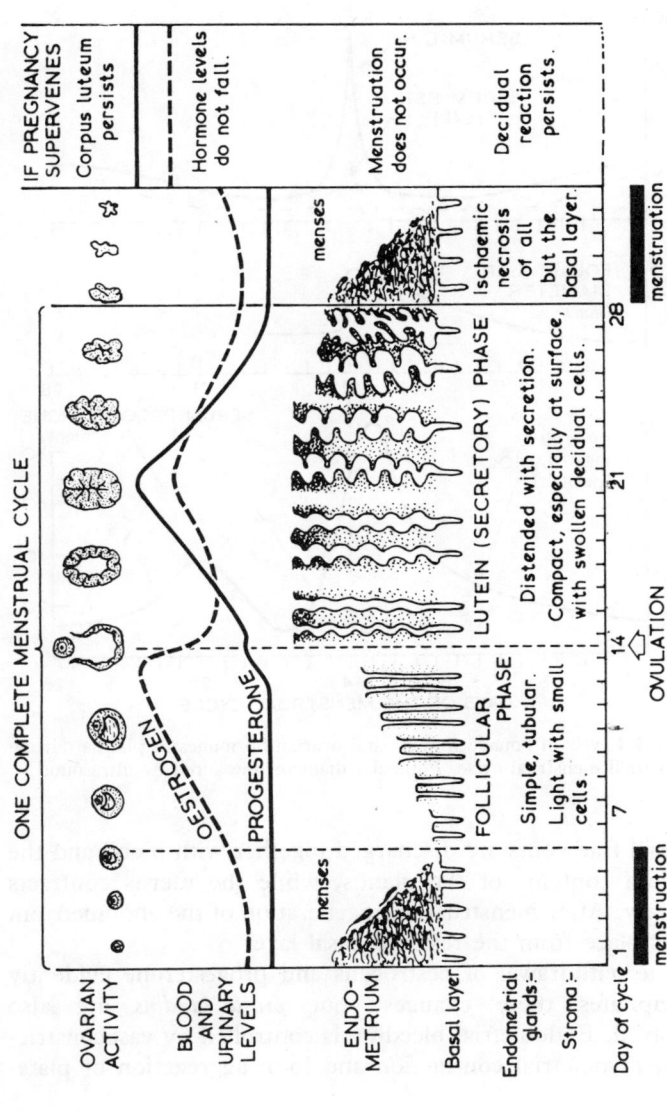

Fig. 1.2 Menstrual cycle.

10 NORMAL FUNCTION

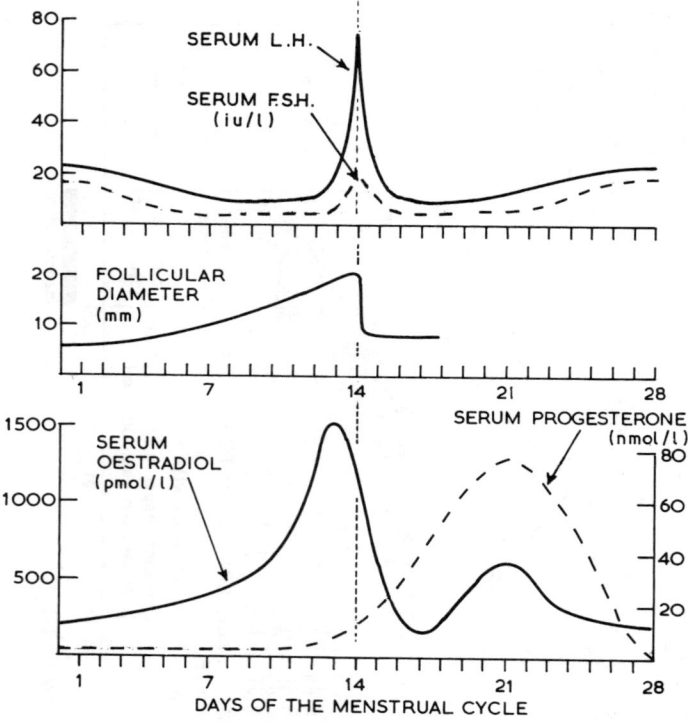

Fig. 1.3 Levels of gonadotrophins and ovarian hormones in plasma during the normal menstrual cycle. Follicular diameter measured by ultrasound.

metrial fragments are discharged together with blood and the mucoid contents of the glands, while the uterus contracts actively. After menstruation regeneration of the endometrium takes place from the residual basal layer.

The withdrawal of oestrogens and progesterone evidently precipitates these changes, but *prostaglandins* are also involved. Endometrial bleeding is controlled by vasoconstriction, myometrial contraction and local aggregation of platelets. Prostaglandins are synthesized in the endometrium and myometrium. $PGF_{2\alpha}$ causes myometrial contraction and vasoconstriction, and is the prostaglandin chiefly concerned in the arrest of menstrual bleeding. PGE_2 and prostacyclin are vasodilators.

Endocrine control of the menstrual cycle

There is a critical and complex interrelation between the levels of pituitary gonadotrophins and ovarian steroids.

On the basis of animal experiments the hypothalamus is believed to contain two centres for releasing hormone. The *tonic centre* is situated just above the pituitary. A moderate rise of oestradiol levels, as seen between the 7th and 10th days of the cycle, inhibits this centre (negative feedback) so that less GnRH is liberated, and the level of FSH falls slightly. The *cyclic centre* is situated above the optic chiasma. A large rise in oestradiol levels, as seen after the 10th day of the cycle, stimulates this centre (positive feedback) to liberate GnRH, and there is a tremendous surge of secretion of FSH and LH. Ovulation occurs about 30 hours after this surge. Both FSH and LH are necessary for normal ovulation and corpus luteum activity.

The granulosa cells of the ripening follicle secrete oestradiol in increasing amounts from the 5th day of the cycle until ovulation. Shortly before ovulation the level of oestradiol falls, but then rises again; and when the corpus luteum is formed there is a rapid rise in levels of progesterone, reaching a peak at about the 20th day.

If pregnancy does not occur in this cycle the corpus luteum regresses and the steroid levels fall about 5 days before menstrual bleeding starts.

With this fall in oestradiol and progesterone levels there is a slight rise in FSH levels, which continues for the first 5 days of the *next* cycle. The cause of this rise is uncertain, but it is necessary for the priming of a number of ovarian follicles. In a normal cycle only one of these follicles undergoes complete maturation and ovulation; we do not know why only one is chosen.

Emotion such as fear, or sexual stimuli, may alter the rhythm, presumably by nervous stimuli acting on the hypothalamus, and so in turn on the pituitary gland.

Clinical features of menstruation

The menstrual discharge over a whole period mesures 30–80 ml, but only half of this is blood; mucus predominates in early and late stages. Clots are unusual as they are liquefied by endometrial fibrolysins unless the bleeding is too heavy for this to occur. Many healthy women have symptoms such as emotional tension, pelvic discomfort and slight frequency just before or during menstruation; but severe or incapacitating pain must be regarded as abnormal. Slight breast enlargement and tenderness are common. Psychological factors certainly accentuate menstrual complaints, but there is objective evidence of metabolic changes; for example temperature rise, and gain of weight due to retention of water and sodium chloride. The term *premenstrual tension* is used for such symptoms (see p. 315).

Menstrual hygiene

Girls should be brought up to regard menstruation as a normal function, during which there should be no cessation of normal activity, bathing or washing. The menstrual discharge is absorbed on an external sanitary towel which is sterilized during commercial manufacture, or on a sterile tampon made of compressed absorbent material which is inserted into the vagina.

An exceedingly rare complication of the use of tampons is

'toxic shock syndrome', characterized by fever, circulatory collapse, diarrhoea and a scarlatiniform rash, attributed to endotoxins produced by certain strains of *Staphylococcus aureus* which may proliferate in the tampons. It is so rare that it would not be justifiable to condemn the use of tampons.

Cyclical changes in the lower genital tract

The normal thick white vaginal secretion is highly acid (pH 5). In response to oestrogens the stratified cells accumulate glycogen, which is converted to lactic acid by Döderlein's bacilli, which are constantly present. The acidity is a barrier against ascending infection, but quickly kills spermatozoa.

The cervical glands secrete an alkaline mucus, which alters in different phases of the menstrual cycle. At midcycle the mucus is less viscous, and spermatozoa can more easily enter it to gain protection from the vaginal acid. Semen contains hyaluronidase, an enzyme that liquefies cervical mucus. Sexual stimulation increases cervical secretion and so may make fertilization more probable, and both cervical and vestibular mucus have a lubricating function in coitus. During coitus there is also a transudate through the vaginal epithelium.

Cyclical changes in the cells of the vaginal epithelium can be shown by staining smears of the desquamated cells.

Sexual maturation

We now return to consider the events which occur at puberty. (The embryology of the female genital organs is described later, on p. 217.)

Pulsatile secretion of GnRH begins before birth and gradually increases towards puberty. Even in the years before puberty FSH and LH levels rise slowly and a few ovarian follicles mature, but oestrogen levels are low. At puberty cyclical release of larger amounts of gonadotrophins begins. Since the pituitary gland and ovaries have functional capacity before puberty the onset of menstruation has been attributed to changing sensitivity of the hypothalamus to feedback from the ovary, described on p. 11. Normal sexual maturation is related to normal nutrition and body weight.

After the first period (the menarche) early cycles may be erratic, but a regular rhythm is soon established.

Puberty

Puberty usually occurs between 12 and 15 years. The whole configuration of the body alters. Skeletal growth slows, female characteristics of the pelvis are accentuated, subcutaneous fat becomes of adult distribution, and the breasts enlarge. Pubic hair appears and the labia majora become larger. The body of the uterus enlarges and now becomes longer than the cervix. Menstruation starts, and other endocrine changes occur, especially shrinkage of the thymus.

The menopause

Endocrine changes at the end of the reproductive period are almost the reverse of those at puberty. The ovarian response ceases, first by failure of ovulation so that progesterone is no longer produced by the ovary, and eventually all ovarian oestrogenic activity ceases. For a time the output of gonadotrophins increases, but finally that too diminishes.

The ovaries atrophy, and the uterus shrinks to a length of about 2 cm, the vaginal portion becoming especially shortened so as to become flush with the vaginal vault. The muscle is largely replaced by fibrous tissue, and the endometrium becomes a thin layer with scanty glands. The vagina narrows and vaginal acidity falls; the labia shrink and pubic hair is lost.

The cessation of menstruation is termed the menopause and usually occurs between 45 and 50 years, though sometimes earlier or later. The commonest event is a gradual increase in the interval between periods, with diminishing loss at each successive period; but sometimes menstruation ceases abruptly. Although common, *any excessive or irregular loss must be regarded as pathological* and investigated. Transient depression and emotional instability are common, libido may be reduced, but is not usually completely lost. 'Hot flushes' (intermittent vasodilatation of the face and trunk) may occur. Weight is sometimes gained.

For the treatment of menopausal symptoms see p. 316.

2

Normal pregnancy

Fertilization and embedding of the embryo

During coitus large numbers of motile spermatozoa are deposited in the upper vagina. Many enter the cervical mucus and ascend into the uterus, but only a few reach the tube, where conjugation of one of them with the oöcyte occurs. The zygote reaches the uterine cavity about 5 days after ovulation, and it will then have started to divide actively. The outermost cells of the embryo (*trophoblast*) are able to digest the superficial cells of the endometrium, so that it buries itself in the thickness of the secretory endometrium, which is now called the *decidua*. Figure 2.1 shows an early pregnancy.

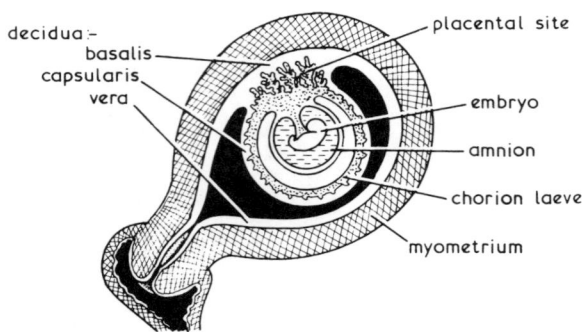

Fig. 2.1 Diagram to show embedding of embryo in decidua.

The trophoblast becomes arranged in two layers — a deep layer of cuboidal cells (cytotrophoblast) and a superficial syncytium (syncytiotrophoblast). These two layers of trophoblast, together with an underlying layer of fetal mesenchyme, constitute the chorion, which gives rise to numerous *chorionic villi*.

Chorionic gonadotrophic hormone

The chorion produces chorionic gonadotrophin (hCG) which resembles LH in its action, and prevents regression of the corpus luteum. hCG is excreted in maternal urine, and the ordinary immunological tests for pregnancy depend upon its presence there. During pregnancy the corpus luteum continues to secrete oestrogen and progesterone, which maintain the decidua. After the first 10 weeks the corpus luteum is no longer essential for maintenance of the pregnancy, as these two hormones are then directly produced by the placenta.

The placenta

At first the embryo is completely surrounded by chorionic villi, but by the 12th week only the villi at the future site of the placenta remain. These villi proliferate to form the placenta, and the remainder of the chorion persists as the *chorionic membrane*.

The fetus soon develops its heart and blood vessels, and some of these vessels extend out of its body along the umbilical cord to the placenta.

The majority of the chorionic villi branch freely in the intervillous space, but a few are attached to maternal decidua (Fig. 2.2). Maternal blood fills the spaces between the villi but does not mix with the fetal blood in the vessels in the villi, although if small injuries to the villi occur a few fetal

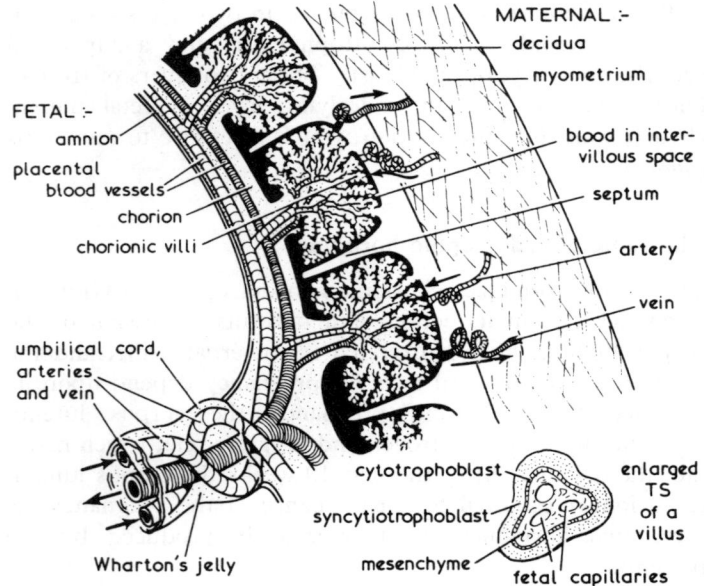

Fig. 2.2 Diagram to show structure of placenta. In reality the villi are far more complex and branched.

red cells or fragments of villi may enter the maternal circulation.

In general the trophoblast and the epithelium of the villi form a semipermeable membrane, preventing the passage of substances of high molecular weight and particles such as bacteria, although some organisms (e.g. those of rubella, syphilis and toxoplasmosis) will invade the fetus. Blood gases and most substances of molecular weight less than 1000 pass freely, but the trophoblast has some selective activity. IgG gammaglobulins and some antibodies of high molecular weight (e.g. rhesus antibodies) reach the fetus. Oestrogens, androgens, cortisone and thyroxine pass the placenta; insulin does not. Most drugs, antibiotics and anaesthetic agents will pass.

The placenta secretes chorionic gonadotrophin (p. 17), oestrogens (p. 5) and progesterone, and these hormones maintain the decidua and cause growth of the uterus and breasts. It also secretes corticotrophin and large amounts of lactogen. The function of the latter is uncertain, but it has prolactin-like and growth-hormone-like activity. Little transfer to the fetus occurs.

The placenta is normally attached to the upper uterine segment. At term it weighs about 500 g and is about 20 cm in diameter. Sometimes the placenta has two lobes, and if one lobe is small and separate (*succenturiate lobe*) it may be retained when the rest of the placenta is delivered and cause postpartum haemorrhage.

The umbilical cord and membranes

The umbilical cord at term is usually about 50 cm long. It contains two arteries and one vein embedded in gelatinous mesodermal tissue (*Wharton's jelly*). When one artery is absent the fetus sometimes shows other abnormalities. The cord is normally attached to the centre of the placenta, but sometimes joins the edge (*battledore insertion*). Rarely the umbilical vessels branch and run on the membranes before reaching the placenta (*velamentous insertion*), and if such a vessel lies below the presenting part (*vasa praevia*) it may be torn during labour.

The uterine cavity at term is lined by maternal decidua, and within that by *chorion*, a thick membrane (of which the placenta is a specialized part), and thin *amnion*. The amnion covers the placenta and umbilical cord, and is continuous with the fetal skin at the navel (Fig. 2.2). The amniotic cavity contains about 1200 ml of *liquor amnii*.

Fetal circulation

The two umbilical arteries carry blood to the placenta and are branches of the hypogastric (internal iliac) arteries. The umbilical vein returns oxygenated blood from the placenta to the portal vein, but much of this blood bypasses the liver through the *ductus venosus* to the inferior vena cava. The lungs are not functioning, and the pulmonary circulation is largely bypassed by two connections between the right and left sides of the circulation:

1. The *foramen ovale* between the two atria.
2. The *ductus arteriosus* between the pulmonary artery and aorta. When the cord is tied and respiration starts the pulmonary circulation opens up, and the foramen ovale and ductus arteriosus close.

Changes in maternal physiology

During pregnancy the uterus grows from a weight of about 60 g to 1000 g by proliferation and enlargement of the smooth muscle cells. The uterine blood vessels are enormously hypertrophied. Especially in the middle layer the muscle fibres are arranged in interlacing bundles which compress the large vascular sinuses when they contract, and so control bleeding after delivery.

The cervix and vagina become so vascular that they are softer and bluish in colour. The cervical glands proliferate and are so distended that the cervix appears to contain a plug of mucus.

The glandular structures of the breasts proliferate in response to oestrogens and progesterone.

During pregnancy the maternal basal metabolic rate increases by about 20%, but in spite of that more weight is gained than is accounted for by the growth of the fetal tissues, the uterus and the breasts. The average gain is 11 kg. The rate of gain is greatest in late pregnancy, when it is about 0.5 kg per week. Part of the gain is water, and the blood volume increases, so that haemodilution occurs and the haemoglobin concentration falls, but there is also a substantial gain in fat reserves.

The cardiac output rises by about 30%, reaching this level by the 28th week and so continuing to term. Peripheral vasodilatation occurs. There is often breathlessness, but the pulmonary vital capacity is not reduced.

The renal threshold for glucose often falls, so that sugar may be found in the urine although the blood sugar is normal (see p. 104). Dilatation of the renal pelves and ureters occurs, but there is no diminution of renal function.

SYMPTOMS AND SIGNS OF PREGNANCY

Duration of pregnancy

The average duration of normal pregnancy is 282 days from the first day of the last menstrual period, i.e., 268 days from ovulation. The expected date of delivery can be estimated by adding seven days to the date of the LMP and subtracting three calendar months.

Symptoms and signs of normal pregnancy

Amenorrhoea

Pregnancy is the commonest cause of amenorrhoea during the child-bearing years. Slight bleeding may occur in early pregnancy, but such bleeding is unrelated to menstruation and should be regarded as abnormal, although often no harm results.

22 NORMAL FUNCTION

Morning sickness

Nausea or vomiting, usually only in the early morning, are common symptoms between the 6th and 14th weeks.

Breast changes

At 6–8 weeks fullness and discomfort may be noted. In brunettes the areolae of the nipples become pigmented at about the 12th week; this change is permanent. Pigmentation may extend to skin beyond the areola (*secondary areola*) at about the 20th week; this will disappear after delivery. Areolar sebaceous glands become active (*Montgomery's tubercles*) and the nipples become more prominent. Clear secretion can be expressed at the 12th week and yellow colostrum near term. Once lactation has occured slight secretion may persist, so that this sign is only useful in the diagnosis of a first pregnancy.

Changes in the skin

In some women stretching of the skin of the abdomen, and less often over the breasts, causes red lines (*striae gravidarum*). These persist but become white after delivery. There may be pigmentation in the midline of the abdomen (*linea nigra*) or on the face (*chloasma uterinum*): these signs will disappear after delivery.

Frequency of micturition

This may occur in early pregnancy because of pressure on the bladder by the uterus in the pelvis.

Changes in the vagina and cervix

These structures become so vascular that they appear blue

NORMAL PREGNANCY 23

and feel soft. There is an increase in vaginal secretion which may cause pruritus vulvae. The uterine isthmus softens before the lower cervix, so that on bimanual examination at about the 9th week the body and cervix of the uterus may feel as if they are separate structures (Hegar's sign).

Enlargement of the uterus

The body of the uterus becomes globular by about the 12th week, and it then rises up into the abdomen. Subsequently the fundus reaches the level of the umbilicus at the 24th week and the xiphoid cartilage at the 36th week. If the fetal head engages in the pelvic cavity the fundus may then descend a little ('lightening'). Painless uterine contractions occur and can be felt during pregnancy.

Clinical signs due to the presence of the fetus

Fetal movements are usually felt by the mother ('quickening') at the 20th week, and may be felt later by the attendant. *Fetal heart sounds* can usually be heard with a fetal stethoscope at the 24th week. Occasionally a *uterine souffle* (a murmur due to blood flow in the uterine vessels) or a *funic souffle* (due to blood flow in umbilical vessels) may be heard with a stethoscope.

Internal ballottement is a sign found on vaginal examination at about the 20th week, when the fetus may float upward in the liquor and then return to tap on the examining finger.

The various parts of the fetus can be felt and recognized by abdominal palpation in late pregnancy, and *external ballottement* may then be possible, when the fetal head can be displaced and then felt to return with a sharp tap. At this time fetal parts can also be distinguished on vaginal examination.

Other symptoms

Other common symptoms include vagaries of appetite, a dislike for smoking, constipation, and breathlessness towards term. Backache is common, but not always due to the pregnancy.

Laboratory tests

During pregnancy large amounts of chorionic gonadotrophin are secreted by the placenta and excreted in the maternal urine. A simple rapid pregnancy test can be performed on a glass slide in the clinic. Human gonadotrophin has antigenic properties, and on injection into animals antisera are produced. The steps of a typical test are:

1. Patient's urine is mixed with anti-hCG. If she is pregnant the urine contains hCG which neutralizes the anti-hCG.
2. The mixture is added to a suspension of particles coated with hCG.
3. If the patient is pregnant there is no reaction because the anti-hCG has been neutralized; if she is *not* pregnant the particles are agglutinated by the unfixed anti-hCG.

Such tests are only reliable 10 days after the first day of the last period, but pregnancy can be diagnosed immediately after a missed period by the more sensitive but more complex radio immunoassay of β-hCG in blood.

Radiological appearance

Fetal bones can be seen in a radiograph from the 16th week, but because of radiation hazards this method is not employed for the diagnosis of pregnancy.

NORMAL PREGNANCY 25

Ultrasonic diagnosis

If sound waves of high frequency are directed through the body they are reflected at any interface between tissues of different physical properties. The returning waves permit echo sounding, so that the depth of interfaces can be measured. In the original A scan the degree of deflection of a dot

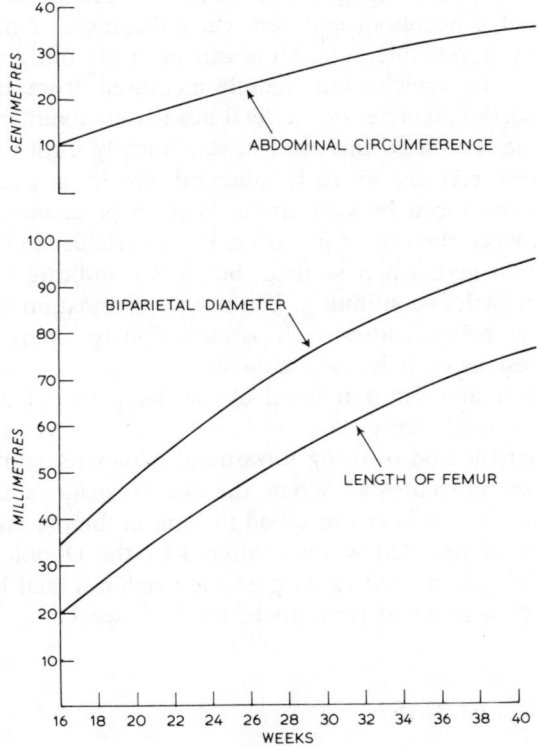

Fig. 2.3 Fetal measurement by ultrasound.

of light on a screen indicated the strength of echo and this allowed measurement of distances between reflecting surfaces. In B scan the brightness of the dot varies according to the strength of echo, and by swinging the beam to and fro across the field a picture like that on a radar screen can be built up. In modern 'real time' machines a linear array or a rotating sector scan gives a continuous image resembling that of a television screen.

With ultrasound the gestation sac can be recognized within 5 weeks of conception, and very early diagnosis of multiple pregnancy is possible. The fetus can be made out from the 6th week, its crown-rump length measured from the 8th week, and the diameter of the fetal head from about the 12th week. The fetal head increases in size linearly until the 30th week, and records of early observations in a case with doubtful dates can be very useful later in pregnancy. After the 30th week the rate of growth is more variable, so that the scan cannot give a precise date, but it will indicate whether normal growth is continuing. Ultrasonic examination can also show fetal abnormalities such as anencephaly, spina bifida, cardiac lesions or polycystic kidneys.

The best and safest method of localizing the placenta is with ultrasound (see p. 90).

Another method of using ultrasound allows recognition of fetal heart movements. When the waves strike a moving object such as the heart, or blood flowing in the placenta, the frequency of reflected waves is altered by the Doppler principle. With simple and easily portable machines fetal life can thus be demonstrated from about the 12th week.

ANTENATAL CARE

Good antenatal care reduces mortality and morbidity in the mother and fetus. It can only start when the woman thinks that she is pregnant and attends for advice, often after 8 weeks. For many women advice before conception would be useful, and some clinics for *pre-pregnancy counselling* have been set up. Those attending might include:

1. Women with pre-existing and continuing disease, e.g. heart disease, hypertension and renal disease diabetes, epilepsy, haemoglobinopathy or any other cause of ill-health. Some of these patients will need advice because they are receiving drugs.
2. Women with a family history of disease or fetal abnormality needing genetic advice.
3. Women who have had an unsuccessful pregnancy from any cause.

Antenatal care includes:

1. *Detection and treatment of any intercurrent illness*. Some disorders begin before the pregnancy, other only arise or are discovered during it.
2. *Detection and treatment of complications of pregnancy*, e.g. antepartum haemorrhage, hypertension, pyelonephritis, anaemia or twins.
3. *Anticipation of complications of labour*, e.g. disproportion or malpresentations.
4. *Fetal considerations* include any foreseeable risk of fetal abnormality, e.g. placental insufficiency, preterm labour or haemolytic disease.
5. *Psychological preparation* for labour and instruction in the care of the baby.

A regular routine is essential. The mother's age, race, parity and social background are all important in obstetrics. At the first visit a *general medical history* is taken, including questions about cardiac disease, tuberculosis, diabetes, infection of the urinary tract and smoking habits.

Any *previous obstetric history* is recorded, including for each pregnancy:

1. Any complications during pregnancy.
2. Method of delivery and any complications, with the weight of the child.
3. Any complications of the puerperium or infant feeding.

A woman who has had four previous pregnancies is often called a grand multipara. Such a patient tends to be older, and if her social conditions are poor she may have anaemia or poor nutrition. Because of the laxity of the uterus malpresentations may occur such as a transverse lie, uterine action may be weak during labour, and there is a risk of postpartum haemorrhage. After the age of 40 there is also an increased risk of Down's syndrome (p. 186).

The *history of the present pregnancy* is then taken, including the date of the last menstrual period, the regularity of previous cycles and (if applicable) the date of discontinuation of oral contraception.

General examination includes examination of the heart, lungs, breasts, legs and teeth. At the first visit a midstream specimen of urine is collected for bacterial culture. The urine is also examined for sugar and protein. If protein is found at any time a midstream specimen is taken to avoid vaginal contamination, and is examined for pus cells and organisms. The blood pressure is recorded, and blood is taken for haemoglobin estimation, grouping, and serological tests for syphilis and rubella antibodies. If the blood group is rhesus negative the blood is examined for Rh antibodies. Coombs' test is a non-specific test for other antibodies. For Negro patients the haemoglobin type is determined by electrophoresis. In many clinics the serum is routinely tested for alphafetoprotein (p. 186). A radiograph of the chest is taken if there is any suspicion of disease.

At *abdominal examination* the size of the uterus is noted, and in later pregnancy the position of the fetus and the fetal heart sounds. A *pelvic examination* is made to exclude any gross abnormality of the bony pelvis or pelvic organs. A cervical smear is taken for examination for cancer cells.

An early *ultrasonic examination* will confirm pregnancy and discover twins, and examination after the 16th week will establish the maturity and exclude many fetal abnormalities.

Antenatal attendances should be monthly until the 30th week, fortnightly until the 36th week and then weekly, but not all these need be to the hospital clinic. Care can be shared with the general practitioner and many examinations can be made by midwives. Most women are booked for hospital delivery, and might be seen there for their initial visit, and then at about the 30th, 36th and 40th weeks, and thereafter if pregnancy is prolonged. Patients with abnormalities may need to be seen more often.

At each visit the urine is examined for protein and sugar, and the blood pressure is taken. The woman is weighed to detect excessive fluid retention, and any oedema is noted. In the later weeks abdominal palpation is performed to find the fetal position and to exclude disproportion (see p. 129). The vaginal examination may be repeated at the 36th week, as it is then easier to assess the size of the pelvic cavity than it is in early pregnancy.

The haemoglobin concentration is estimated again at the 30th week and repeatedly if there is anaemia, and further antibody tests are done if the group is rhesus negative.

The full description of the fetal position includes the *lie* (longitudinal, oblique or transverse), *attitude* (flexed or extended, especially of the head), *presentation* (vertex, face, brow, breech or shoulder) and *position* (of the presenting part relative to the pelvis, e.g. left occipito-posterior position). (see Fig. 2.4).

The fetal heart sounds are usually heard through the back

30 NORMAL FUNCTION

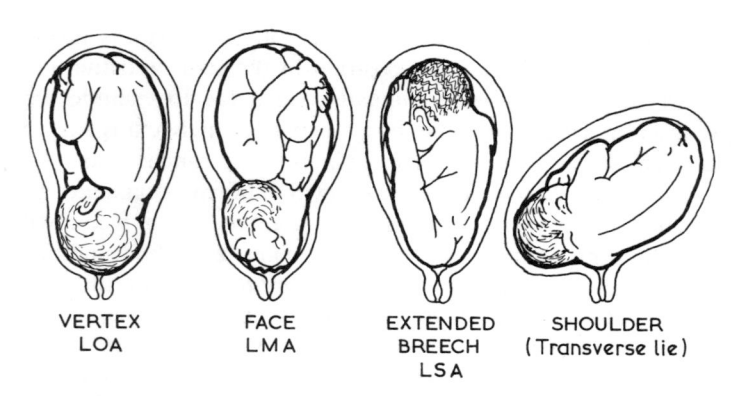

| VERTEX LOA | FACE LMA | EXTENDED BREECH LSA | SHOULDER (Transverse lie) |

Fig. 2.4 Fetal presentation, position, attitude and lie.

of the fetus, and lower in the maternal abdomen with a vertex than with a breech presentation.

The presenting part of the fetus is said to be *engaged* if its widest diameter has entered the pelvic brim. The height of the fundus above the symphysis pubis is measured, and the distance in centimetres normally corresponds with the duration of gestation in weeks until descent and engagement of the presenting part occurs.

The size of the fetus should, as far as possible, be assessed by careful palpation at each antenatal examination after the 28th week to detect any fetus that is small-for-dates (see p. 197). If there is any doubt about the rate of fetal growth repeated ultrasonic measurement of the circumference of the fetal abdomen, the biparietal diameter and the length of the femur are made.

If the fetal welfare is in doubt the mother may be asked to note the activity of the fetus, perhaps by counting the number of kicks felt during 1 hour each day. A record of the fetal heart rate may also be made with an abdominal ultrasonic receiver over 30 minutes. The normal fetus has spells of activity during which the heart rate shows variation, and the rate also responds to uterine contractions. If growth is defective, or fetal activity is abnormal, the case should be reviewed for any possible cause of placental insufficiency or fetal abnormality.

Advice to the patient

It is convenient to give each patient a booklet as well as verbal directions.

Diet. An adequate intake of protein is needed (meat, fish, eggs, cheese). If fresh fruit and milk (1 pint daily) are added most vitamins and minerals will be adequately provided, but tablets containing ferrous fumarate (300 mg daily) and folic acid (300 micrograms daily) are given routinely.

Alcohol and *smoking* should be strongly discouraged.

Teeth. Any carious teeth should be filled, and oral sepsis treated.

Bowels. Constipation is common and senna is effective.

Coitus. Coitus is unwise if there has been any bleeding, and in the last month.

Exercise. Exercise should be taken regularly, but over-fatigue avoided.

Breasts. Application of spirit or lanolin is useless; daily washing is all that is needed. If the nipples are flat, cups ('shells') may be worn under the brassière to press on the areolae.

Psychological preparation

Pregnant women may have many anxieties relating to health, labour, the unborn child and family relationships. Although 'old wives' tales are now less common, the press and television sometimes exaggerate problems and cause new anxieties.

Ideal antenatal care would give time to deal with each individual patient's anxieties, but in the rush of hospital work this may be impossible and then antenatal mothercraft classes are invaluable, at which questions should be encouraged and carefully answered. The patient's general practitioner and midwife can play an important role in advising her.

In spite of loud claims, there is no scientific evidence that the course or safety of labour is altered by any form of antenatal exercises, although these may give confidence to those who believe in them.

If it is intended that the husband is to be with his wife during labour he should also be given preparatory instruction.

Selection of patients for hospital care

Although it is often claimed that it is as safe to have a baby at home as in hospital this is untrue, and reports which claim to show this are derived from groups of patients who are highly selected, both obstetrically and socially. The risk, especially to the fetus, is greatly increased if an emergency arises at home during labour and the patient then has to be removed to hospital. If hospital beds are limited the following patients should have priority:

1. *Primigravidae*, who have an increased risk of hypertension, prolonged labour and operative delivery, and a relatively high perinatal mortality. The very young or the elderly primigravida needs special care.
2. *Grand multiparae*. After the fourth pregnancy the maternal risk exceeds that of a first pregnancy. The patients are older, and postpartum and antepartum haemorrhage, malpresentations and fetal abnormalities are more common.
3. Patients with a *history of obstetric abnormality* which may recur, such as hypertension, disproportion, and postpartum haemorrhage or the presence of a Caesarean scar.

NORMAL PREGNANCY

4. Patients with *intercurrent medical disorders*, such as cardiac disease.
5. Patients who are found to have any obstetric abnormality in the current pregnancy, such as twins, antepartum haemorrhage or a malpresentation will require hospital treatment, but such abnormalities may not be evident at the time of booking.
6. If it is possible that a paediatric problem will arise it is essential that delivery should take place in a hospital with a fully equipped neonatal care unit.

General practitioners who have had basic obstetric experience, such as that gained in a 6 months resident hospital obstetric appointment, may share antenatal care with the hospital clinic, and many patients can be delivered in G.P. obstetric units, provided that there is good liaison with, and close proximity to, specialist obstetric and paediatric services, and that patients with foreseeable abnormalities are not accepted.

3

Normal labour

During pregnancy painless uterine contractions occur. When labour begins the contractions become stronger, more frequent and more regular, and painful. The pain is caused by ischaemia as each contraction arrests the myometrial blood flow. At the onset of labour the membranes over the internal os separate slightly and there is a little bleeding and discharge of mucus from the cervical canal (the '*show*'). Sometimes, especially if the presenting part does not fit well into the pelvic cavity, the membranes rupture early in labour.

The uterus has two functional divisions. The *lower segment* consists of the cervix and the lowest part of the body of the uterus. The rest is the *upper segment*, and this contracts more strongly than the lower segment so that the latter is gradually stretched and becomes thinner. The junction between the thick upper segment and the thin lower segment is *Bandl's retraction ring* (Fig. 3.1).

The **cause of the onset of normal labour** is still uncertain. In sheep at term the fetal anterior pituitary secretes ACTH which causes the fetal adrenal cortex to liberate glucocorticoids which play a part in initiating labour. It is uncertain whether this is true for the human fetus, although pregnancy may be prolonged with anencephalic fetuses with abnormal adrenal cortices.

The evidence is against initiation of labour by oxytocin from the maternal or fetal posterior pituitary glands.

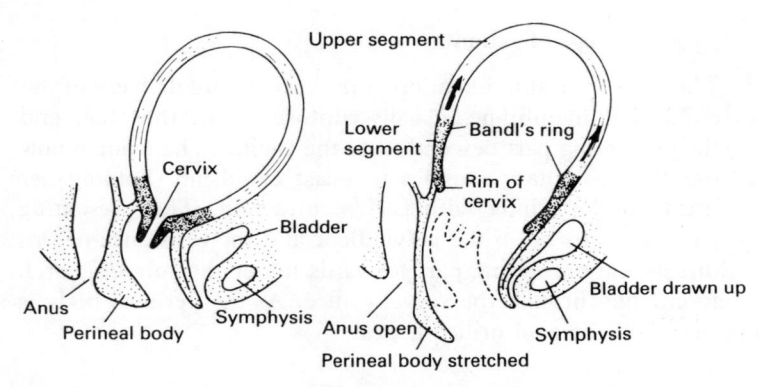

Fig. 3.1 Changes in uterus, vagina, perineum and adjacent structures during labour.

Placental progesterone may inhibit uterine activity during pregnancy, perhaps by blocking release of prostaglandin. At term high levels of oestradiol may stimulate release of prostaglandins from the myometrium and decidua.

The sensitivity of the myometrium to oxytocin or prostaglandins, or to stretching, increases as pregnancy approaches term. Over-stretching of the uterus (e.g., by twins) may cause premature labour, and rupture of the membranes will induce labour in late pregnancy.

First stage of labour

This lasts until the cervix is fully dilated. During this stage the lower segment and cervix are drawn up over the contents of the uterus so that the cervix is first shortened ('taken-up') and then dilated (see Fig. 3.1). As the supravaginal cervix is drawn up the bladder is carried up with it to become an abdominal organ. Between contractions the upper segment muscle fibres retain their tone, so that the fibres do not relax completely and any advance is held (*retraction*).

Second stage of labour

This lasts from full dilatation of the cervix until delivery of the child. The membranes usually rupture during this stage and the presenting part descends into the vagina. The woman now uses her voluntary muscles to assist expulsion, holding her breath and pushing with each contraction. The presenting part descends on to the pelvic floor and the resistance of this directs the presenting part forwards under the subpubic arch to emerge through the vulval orifice. As the perineal body is stretched the anal orifice gapes.

Third stage of labour

After delivery of the child the uterus contracts to separate and expel the placenta and membranes, and then continues to contract strongly enough to compress the large uterine sinuses and prevent bleeding until the blood in them clots. Separation of the placenta occurs by splitting of the decidual layer.

THE BONY PELVIS

To understand the mechanism of labour and the complications which can arise it is necessary to have some knowledge of the shape and size of the pelvic cavity and of the size of the fetus. The normal dimensions of the pelvis will be given, but in a particular case all that matters is the size of the fetus relative to that of the pelvis. For obstetric purposes only the cavity of the pelvis, extending from the pelvic brim to the pelvic outlet, need be considered.

The pelvic brim

The plane of the brim is inclined at about 60° to the horizontal. It is bounded by a line running from the sacral promontory, along the sacral ala, across the sacro-iliac joint, and along the ilio-pectineal line and pubic crest to the back of the symphysis pubis (Fig. 3.2). The normal antero-posterior diameter (*true conjugate*) is 11 cm and the normal transverse diameter is 13 cm. In the patient the true conjugate cannot be felt, but in cases of severe pelvic contraction the *diagonal conjugate* (from the lower margin of the

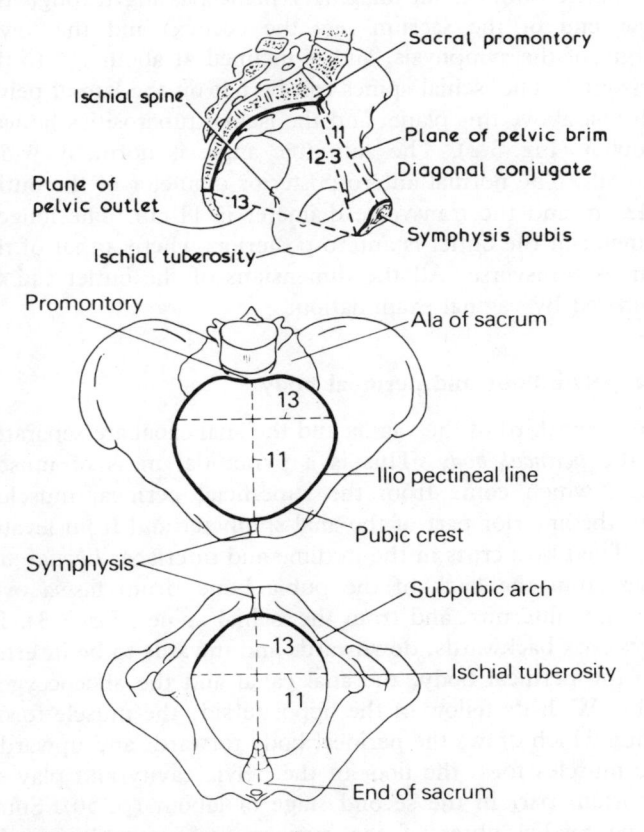

Fig. 3.2 Pelvic measurements (cm).

symphysis to the promontory) may sometimes be determined by digital examination, and the true conjugate measures 1.3 cm less. In late pregnancy the best pelvimeter for the brim is the fetal head.

The pelvic outlet

The pelvic outlet is an imaginary plane passing through the lower end of the sacrum (*not* the coccyx) and the lower margin of the symphysis, and is inclined at about 20° to the horizontal. The ischial spines can be felt on the lateral pelvic wall just above this plane, and the ischial tuberosities lie well below it (Fig. 3.2). The subpubic angle is normally wider than 80°. The normal antero-posterior diameter of the outlet is 13 cm and the transverse diameter is 11 cm. The longest diameter of the outlet is antero-posterior, whereas that of the brim is transverse. All the dimensions of the outlet can be estimated by vaginal examination.

The pelvic floor and perineal body

The lower third of the vagina and the anal canal are separated by the *perineal body*. This is a pyramidal mass of muscle fibres, which come from the superficial perineal muscles, from the anterior part of the anal sphincter and from levator ani. The fibres cross in the midline and interlace. *Levator ani* arises from the back of the pubic bone, from fascia over obturator internus, and from the ischial spine (Fig. 3.3). Its fibres pass backwards, downwards and inwards to be inserted into the perineal body, the anal canal and the anococcygeal raphé. With its fellow of the opposite side the muscle forms a sling which draws the perineal body forwards and upwards. The muscles form the floor of the pelvic cavity and play an important part in the second stage of labour (p. 50). Some of the medial fibres of the muscles are inserted into the

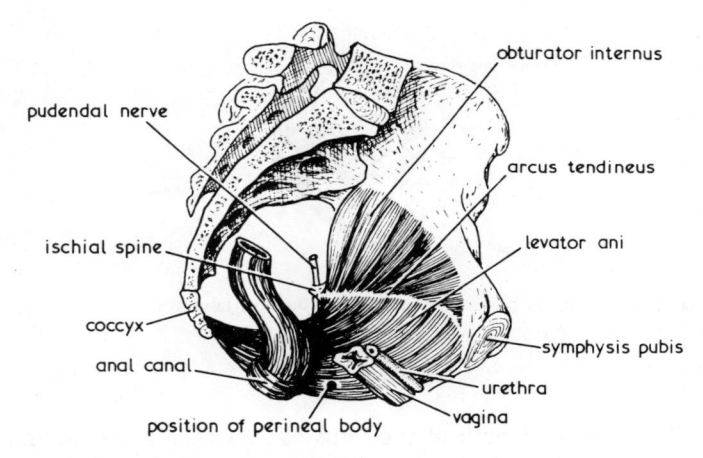

Fig. 3.3 Sagittal section of pelvis to show levator ani muscle.

urethra and may help in maintaining urinary continence, as discussed on p. 353.

FETAL WEIGHT AND MEASUREMENTS

Normal fetuses vary considerably in weight, but as a rough guide the following table is given:

24 weeks	700 g
28 weeks	1100 g
32 weeks	1500 g
36 weeks	2500 g
40 weeks	3500 g

The fetus may be small in cases of multiple pregnancy, with some malformations, in cases of placental insufficiency, especially those associated with hypertension or renal disease, and if the mother smokes heavily. The fetus is often overweight in cases of diabetes.

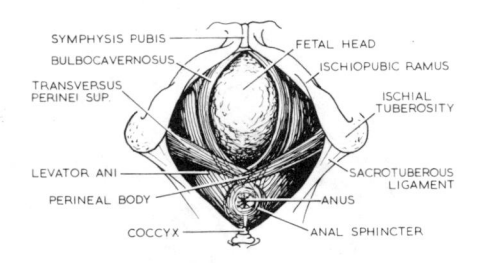

Fig. 3.4 Muscles of pelvic floor in second stage of labour.

The average length of the fetus at 20 weeks is 25 cm and at term is 50 cm.

THE FETAL HEAD

The bones of the vault of the fetal skull are not rigidly fixed together but are mobile at the sutures. The two halves of the frontal bone are still separate, and there are two large membranous fontanelles. During labour moulding of the skull occurs by movement and overriding of the edges of the bones. Terms used in description and the normal measurements of the skull at term are shown in Fig. 3.5. It will be seen that the diameter of engagement is least when the head is fully flexed or fully extended.

The scalp

The periosteum is firmly attached to the edges of the bones, so that a subperiosteal haematoma (*cephalhaematoma*) is confined to one bone. Oedema of the scalp during labour (*caput succedaneum*) is not so confined and lies over the presenting part of the head.

NORMAL LABOUR 41

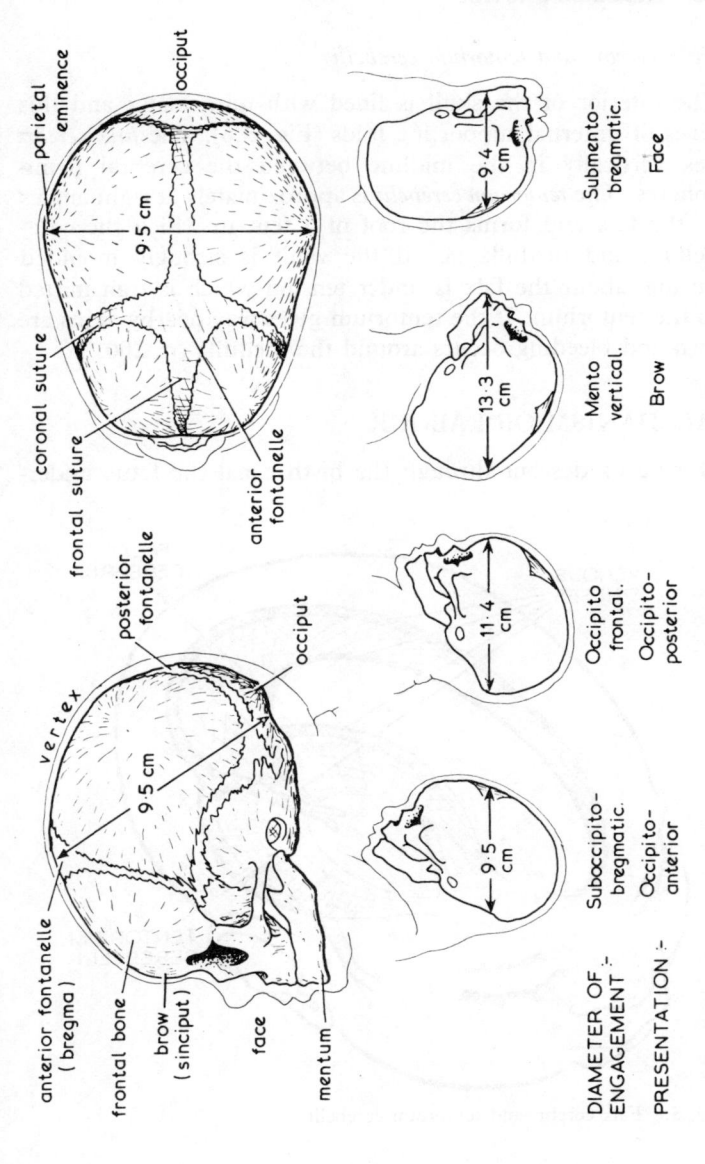

Fig. 3.5 Fetal head.

Falx cerebri and tentorium cerebelli

The interior of the skull is lined with dura mater and this gives off internal supporting folds (Fig. 3.6). The *falx cerebri* lies vertically in the midline between the cerebral hemispheres. The *tentorium cerebelli* is approximately at right angles to the falx and forms the roof of a tent in which the cerebellum and medulla lie. If the vault is strongly moulded during labour the falx is under tension which is transmitted to the tentorium. If the tentorium gives way nearby veins are torn and bleeding occurs around the medulla (p. 200).

MECHANISM OF LABOUR

During its descent through the birth canal the fetus under-

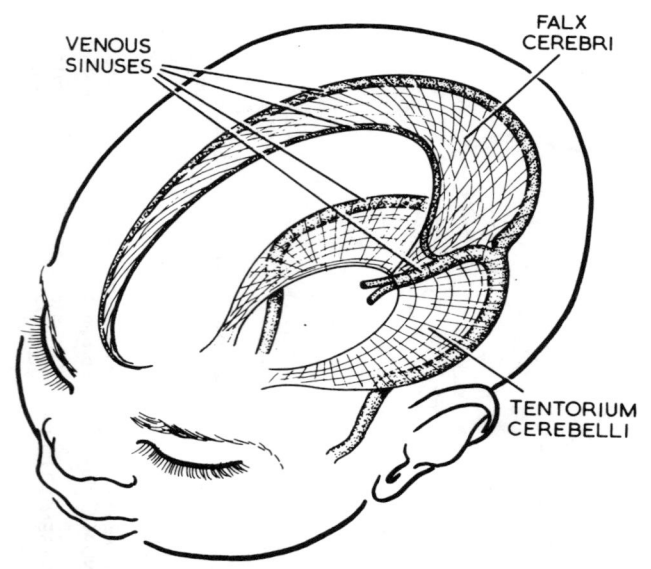

Fig. 3.6 Falx cerebri and tentorium cerebelli.

goes movements which are described as the mechanism of labour. At the onset of labour the head normally lies in the transverse or oblique diameter of the pelvis (Fig. 3.7). As the head descends it becomes more *flexed* so that the occiput becomes the lowest part of the head and impinges on the

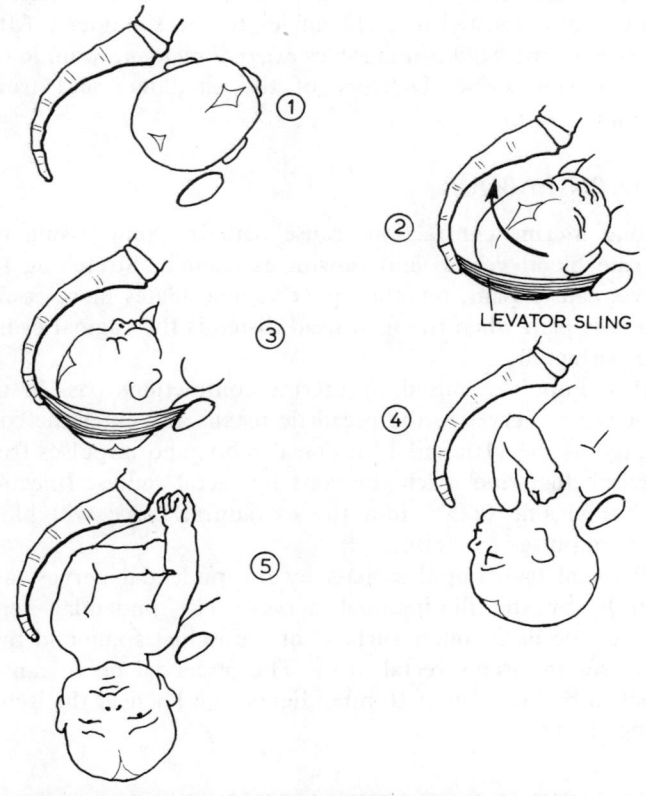

Fig. 3.7 Mechanism of normal labour: (1) flexed head engaged in transverse diameter of pelvis; (2) head has descended into pelvic floor and occiput is rotating forwards; (3) internal rotation complete; (4) birth of head by extension; (5) external rotation of head: shoulders now in anteroposterior diameter of pelvis.

pelvic floor. The two levator ani muscles form a gutter which slopes downwards and forwards in the midline. This gutter directs the occiput forwards, a movement called *internal rotation*. The occiput now passes under the subpubic arch and the head is born by *extension*. The shoulders remain in the anteroposterior diameter of the pelvis as they descend, so that the head is now twisted at right angles to the shoulders. After delivery of the head it undergoes *external rotation*, to undo the twist of the neck. Delivery of the shoulders and trunk follows.

PAIN IN LABOUR

Strong uterine contractions cause pain by compressing the uterine blood vessels and causing ischaemia. Stretching the cervix causes pain, but the upper vagina dilates more easily. There is pain when the fetal head distends the vaginal orifice and perineum.

Pain impulses caused by uterine contractions pass in the hypogastric nerves to the preaortic plexus and enter the cord as high as the 11th and 12th dorsal roots, and impulses from cervical dilatation reach the cord by sacral routes. Injection of bupivicaine 0.25% into the extradural space will block these impulses (p. 180).

Perineal pain impulses pass by the pudendal nerves, and slightly by the ilio-inguinal nerves. The pudendal nerve crosses the back (outer surface) of the ischial spine and then traverses the ischio-rectal fossa. The pudendal nerve can be blocked by injection of 10 ml of lignocaine 1% near the ischial spine (p. 180).

MANAGEMENT OF NORMAL LABOUR

Preparation of the patient

When labour begins the woman should take a bath or shower.

There is no need to shave or clip the vulval hair; there is no evidence that this reduces infection.

General examination

Unless the patient has had regular antenatal care a full obstetric history is taken and general examination is made. In every case the urine is tested, and the blood pressure is recorded throughout labour.

Abdominal examination

This will show whether the presenting part is engaged. The frequency and strength of uterine contractions are assessed. The fetal heart rate is recorded at least half hourly in the first stage of labour and more frequently in the second stage. This may be done with an electronic ratemeter while the uterine contractions are simultaneously recorded with a tocometer (p. 48).

Vaginal examinations

These are required during labour to establish the presentation, to follow the progress of dilatation of the cervix, to discover whether the membranes have ruptured and whether the liquor is clear. The ischial spines are landmarks by which to judge the degree of descent of the presenting part. Vaginal examination is preferable to rectal examination, which gives less accurate information. Vaginal examination is performed routinely at the onset of labour and when the membranes rupture — in the second instance to eliminate the rare possibility of prolapse of the cord. Examinations should be made at least 3-hourly, and more frequently when progress is in doubt.

Prevention of infection

Pathogenic bacteria may be introduced into the genital tract during labour and cause puerperal infection. Coliform bacteria are constantly present on the perineum, and staphylococci and streptococci may be widespread in a hospital, and these and other organisms may be carried on the skin or in the nose or throat of attendants. Gowns should be worn, and sterilized gloves for any examination or operation.

In making a vaginal examination the genitalia are cleansed with swabs moistened with chlorhexidine solution (1:2000) passing each swab once from before backwards. The labia are separated and some chlorhexidine cream is placed around the vaginal orifice, into which the fingers are passed without touching neighbouring areas.

Progress of labour

Accurate records are essential for good obstetrics. The progress of cervical dilatation, the descent of the head, fetal heart rate, administration of drugs and other events in labour can be recorded on a time-sheet called a *partogram*, which is used to monitor the progress of labour. Figure 3.3 shows normal sigmoid curves for a primigravid and for a multigravid patient. There is first a 'latent phase', which is variable in duration but often lasts for about 8 hours from the onset of labour until the cervix is 4–5 cm dilated in a primigravida and 2–3 cm dilated in a multigravida. The 'active phase' follows and lasts for about 3 hours during which the rate of cervical dilatation increases and should be not less than 1 cm per hour. In practical management the patient's partogram is compared with a normal curve; if progress is delayed her curve will be 'to the right' of normal.

Unassisted normal labour is always best and occurs in most

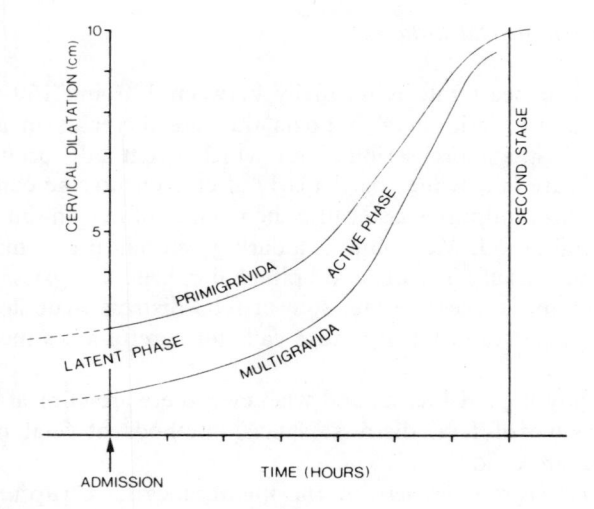

Fig. 3.8 Diagram to show normal progress of cervical dilatation.

cases, but if cervical dilatation does not occur at the normal rate the case needs special management. If examination excludes serious disproportion or malpresentation, labour is augmented by giving an intravenous infusion of 2 units of Syntocinon in 500 ml of normal glucose solution run at 40 drops per minute. The rate the drip is regulated according to the uterine contractions, which must be carefully observed. Fetal death or uterine rupture can occur if the drip is not properly supervised, and the method is only suitable for fully staffed obstetric units, to which patients with delay in labour should be taken. Automatic machines are available which regulate the infusion according to the rate of the contractions recorded by a tocometer, but an ordinary drip can be used so long as the control is accurate. Fetal monitoring is desirable (see below).

Detection of fetal distress

The fetal heart rate is normally between 120 and 160 beats per minute. With fetal hypoxia the rate increases in a few cases, but a more serious sign which eventually occurs in every case is slowing, particularly after each uterine contraction. Vagal impulses also cause the passage of meconium from the fetal bowel. Meconium is a dark green mixture of mucus, bile, intestinal ferments and epithelial debris. The passage of meconium is a less certain sign of fetal distress than slowing of the heart rate, but it always calls for careful assessment of the case.

In any high-risk case, and whenever there are clinical signs suggestive of fetal distress, special methods of fetal monitoring are used.

Fetal heart ratemeters. If the membranes have ruptured a small electrode can be attached to the fetal scalp to monitor the fetal heart rate from ECG signals. Alternatively the fetal heart movements can be monitored through the abdominal and uterine wall with ultrasound. Uterine contractions are recorded on the same trace by an external tocometer which is placed on the abdomen, or with an intra-amniotic catheter to measure intrauterine pressure. 'Dips' in the heart rate may occur with uterine contractions. These decelerations are of little significance if the rate between contractions is normal, if they occur soon after the start of the contractions, and if the rate quickly returns to normal (Fig. 3.9). Decelerations which occur later after the start of the contractions and are prolonged are a warning of fetal danger, especially if there is also bradycardia between contractions. Such a trace would be an indication for taking a sample of fetal blood (see below). The heart rate normally shows a beat-to-beat variation, and this is lost with hypoxia or deep sedation, so that the trace is flat.

Apart from hypoxia, dips in the trace may also be caused by compression of the fetal head.

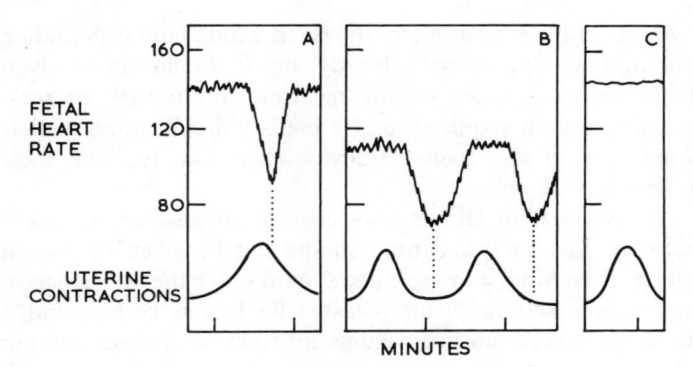

Fig. 3.9 Diagram to show traces obtained with fetal ratemeter; (A) early deceleration occurring soon after uterine contraction; (B) late and prolonged deceleration with basal bradycardia; (C) flat trace with loss of beat-to-beat variation.

Fetal blood sampling. Before any intervention such as Caesarean section the presence of hypoxia must be confirmed by examination of a sample of blood from the fetal scalp. To obtain this a tubular amnioscope is passed through the cervix and, after pricking the scalp, 0.3 ml of blood is collected with a fine heparinized tube. If there is hypoxia carbon dioxide accumulates and the fetal tissues begin anaerobic metabolism with conversion of glycogen to lactic acid, and the pH of the blood falls. The fetus is at risk if the pH lies below 7.20 and delivery with forceps or by Caesarean section is usually necessary. If the pH is below 7.27 a second sample may be taken after 30 minutes to confirm or refute suspected fetal distress.

Normal first stage

During this stage the woman is more comfortable if she is up and about. When contractions become regular and if they cause distress an intramuscular injection of 200 mg of pethidine is given. Other drugs (e.g., promazine 50 mg) may be given in addition or as alternatives. In a long labour pethidine 100 mg may be repeated 2-hourly, but it should not be given if delivery is expected within that time. During labour reassurance is often required, and a patient should never be left alone in a closed room. Many women like to have their husbands with them.

Any woman in labour may require an anaesthetic unexpectedly, and food and fluid should not be given by mouth which, if vomited and aspirated, could enter the air passages. In a long labour the urine is tested for ketone bodies, and if these are present an intravenous infusion of glucose solution is given.

In the first stage progress is assessed by the dilatation of the cervix, which should be thin and well applied to the presenting part. If the membranes remain intact when labour is established they are ruptured with a pair of toothed forceps.

Epidural anaesthesia (p. 180) may be started in this stage, and continued until delivery. Alternatively inhalation analgesia may be used when the first stage is well established (see below).

Normal second stage

It is important that the general atmosphere of the labour room should be calm and quiet. For normal women a 'birthing room' with ordinary domestic furniture may be provided in hospital. During the second stage the woman is kept on her bed, and indeed most women will prefer this. If her trunk is well supported with her head upright, with each contraction she can put her hands behind her knees and push effectively. Some have advocated 'birthing chairs' instead of beds, but if a general anaesthetic is to be given to any patient it is absolutely essential that she should be placed on a bed which can immediately be tilted head-down in an emergency.

In a few women the dorsal position causes 'supine hypotension' because the uterus compresses the inferior vena cava and impedes venous return; if there is fetal distress the patient should be placed on her side.

If the patient desires it, pain may be relieved by an inhalation of nitrous oxide and oxygen. Machines have been devised which only deliver the gas mixture when the patient holds the mask over her face and breathes deeply, and cylinders which contain a mixture of equal parts of nitrous oxide and oxygen (Entonox) are available. In addition a pudendal nerve block (p. 180) or infiltration of the perineum with lignocaine 1% may be used, unless an epidural injection has already been given.

In this stage progress is judged by descent of the presenting part, and eventually by bulging of the perineum.

For delivery sterile towels are arranged and antiseptic cream is freely applied to the vulva. If the bladder is full a catheter is passed.

There are a few patients who demand to be delivered in 'natural' positions, standing, crouching, or on their hands and knees. While their right of choice cannot be denied, it must be explained to them that there is danger to the child if the fetal heart rate is not regularly observed, and that care of the perineum is hardly possible in such positions.

Delivery of the head

To prevent tearing of the perineum the attendant must maintain flexion of the head with his hand until it is crowned (i.e. the parietal eminences are free), and must control the rate of delivery. Once the head is crowned it is delivered slowly between pains when the uterus is relaxed. If the perineum threatens to tear or if there is any delay an episiotomy is performed. The incision starts in the midline and then passes backwards and laterally to avoid the anal sphincter.

Delivery of the shoulders

The perineum is often damaged during delivery of the shoulders and vigilance should not be relaxed at this moment. If a loop of cord is around the neck this is either slipped over the head or clamped and cut.

The head is first drawn towards the sacrum to make sure that the anterior shoulder has passed under the subpubic arch (Fig. 3.10). The head is then drawn towards the symphysis and the posterior shoulder usually sweeps over the perineum. If it does not do so traction is made with a finger in the posterior axilla.

An intravenous or intramuscular injection of Syntocinon is given as soon as the delivery of the shoulders is safely under way (see Third Stage p. 53).

Immediate care of the child

As soon as possible the pharynx is cleared with a mucus aspirator, even before delivery of the shoulders if someone is free to do this. The child is kept at the same level as the placenta in the uterus until the cord ceases to pulsate. The cord is then clamped or tied in two places and then cut at

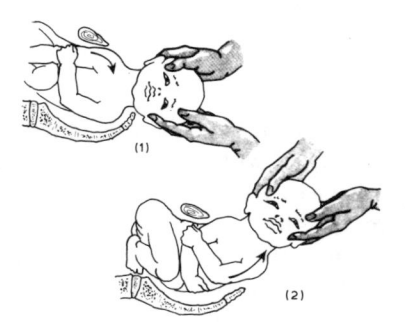

Fig. 3.10 Delivery of shoulders.

least 5 cm from the umbilicus. For the action to be taken if respiration is not immediately established see p. 189. Unless resuscitation is required the baby should at once be given to the mother to see and hold, possibly even before the cord is cut. Le Boyer has stressed the importance of immediate close 'skin to skin' contact between the mother and her baby, which promotes emotional bonding. A normal baby should always be kept closely beside its mother.

Third stage

If no assistance is given in the third stage, the uterus usually remains quiescent for some minutes. It then contracts to separate the placenta completely and to expel it from the upper segment into the dilated lower segment and vagina. With normal retraction of the upper segment the uterine vessels in its wall are compressed and there is only slight bleeding. The patient may be able to expel the placenta from the vagina by contraction of her abdominal muscles.

Signs of separation

When the placenta has separated and the uterus is contracting the fundus feels hard and globular, is mobile from side to side, and rises in the abdomen. The cord lengthens, and there may be a gush of blood, normally of less than 100 ml.

Active management

It is now the general practice to assist the third stage actively, except in cases of hypertension (see below), because this reduces the average blood loss and, more importantly, the number of cases of severe bleeding. Directly the anterior shoulder of the fetus is safely past the subpubic arch, the mother is given Syntocinon 5 units intravenously or intramuscularly. This is perferred to ergometrine (which can be given in the same way in 500 microgram doses) because the latter may cause nausea and vomiting and hypertension.

With either method the uterus contracts strongly and the placenta separates almost at once and is delivered by the *Brandt-Andrews method*. The patient must be in the dorsal position. The attendant stands on her right side and places his left hand just above the symphysis pubis. Upward pressure is maintained with this hand to displace the uterus from the pelvis. (Fig. 3.11) This avoids the risk of inversion while steady downward and backward traction on the cord is made with the other hand. There should be no delay in delivery of the placenta after giving Syntocinon or ergometrine; otherwise there is a slight risk of the placenta being retained by strong contraction of the lower segment.

The Brandt-Andrews manoeuvre is to be distinguished from 'expression' of the placenta by squeezing the fundus

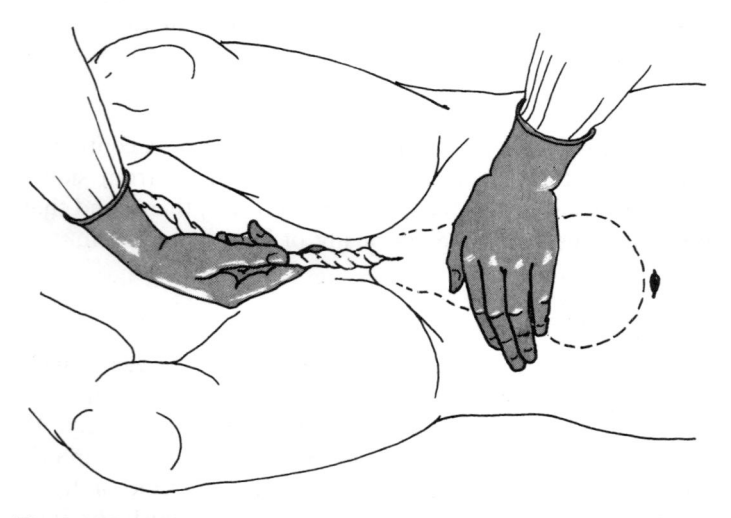

Fig. 3.11 Brandt-Andrews manoeuvre.

violently. This may cause shock, is ineffective, and will cause bleeding if the placenta is only partly separated.

In patients with hypertension Syntocinon or ergometrine is not used unless abnormal bleeding occurs, because there is some risk of increasing the blood pressure and causing postpartum eclampsia. In such cases placental separation is awaited before delivering it by Brandt-Andrews method.

In all cases the placenta and membranes are examined after delivery and the placental weight should be recorded. If any part of the placenta is missing the uterus must be explored. Incomplete membranes are of less consequence. The number of cord vessels should be noted; when one artery is absent there are often fetal abnormalities.

4

Normal puerperium

The puerperium is the period after delivery during which the organs return to their ordinary state. It lasts about 6 weeks.

Involution of the uterus

The large vessels in the uterine wall are occluded with blood clot and a new system of smaller vessels develops by organization of the clot. Rapid autolysis of the muscle cells occurs. After delivery the fundus is about 12 cm above the symphysis, but the uterus becomes impalpable in the abdomen by the 10th day. The uterine cavity decreases rapidly in size, reaching the non-pregnant dimension by about the 7th day. The cervix also becomes closed in this time, and the pelvic floor soon regains its tone.

Lochia

Decidual remnants, except for the basal layer from which regeneration of the endometrium occurs, are discharged in the lochia. At first the discharge chiefly consists of red blood cells, but later it becomes paler and contains more leucocytes. Red lochia continues for at least 14 days. Excessive bleeding occurs when placental tissue is retained. The lochia becomes offensive with some bacterial infections.

Breasts

During pregnancy the ducts and acini of the breasts proliferate. The ducts contain *colostrum*, a yellow fluid containing many fat globules and with a high protein content. Secretion of milk does not occur until after delivery when the hormone *prolactin* is released from the anterior pituitary gland. On the fourth day after delivery acute engorgement of the breasts may occur when secretion begins. Stimulation of the nipple by the infant causes reflex secretion of oxytocin by the posterior pituitary gland, and this not only causes uterine contractions ('*after-pain*') but also contraction of myoepithelial cells around the acini and the consequent outflow of milk.

General metabolic changes

All the changes of pregnancy such as increased metabolic rate, increased cardiac output, fluid retention and changes in the renal tract are quickly reversed, except that most women have gained weight. Some of this is lost during lactation.

MANAGEMENT OF THE NORMAL PUERPERIUM

Prevention of infection

The temperature and pulse rate are recorded as these will give early warning of infection of the genital or urinary tract.

Aseptic technique is continued in the puerperium. Sterilized vulval pads are worn and frequently changed. Vaginal douching is harmful, and vulval 'bathedowns' are of no value in preventing infection. As soon as patients are up they may use a bidet or bath themselves. Nevertheless precautions against cross-infection must be strict, and any infected patient is isolated and her toilet facilities kept separate.

58 NORMAL FUNCTION

Sleep and rest

Undue excitement or insomnia should be treated with hypnotics. In the early puerperium a transient attack of depression, with weeping, is common; it only calls for sympathetic reassurance. More persistent depression or aversion to the baby must be taken more seriously.

Patients with no complications are allowed up within a few hours, but they should have at least 10 days rest from housework. Early ambulation reduces the risk of venous thrombosis without any evident increase in the incidence of prolapse.

Too many visitors should not be allowed. In hospitals children are sometimes excluded because of the risk of infection, but this rule is founded on theory rather than any adverse experience.

In hospital physiotherapists can teach exercises for the abdominal and pelvic floor muscles, which patients may continue at home.

Hospital stay

Provided that the patient's doctor and the community midwife are available to supervise them at home, fit mothers and babies can be discharged after 48 hours or even earlier, although many normal patients stay for 5 to 6 days, which has the advantage that lactation can be established before discharge.

Diet

The same diet as that recommended during pregnancy is appropriate, but abundant fluid is required during lactation.

Bowels

For constipation senna or cascara may be used, or an enema

given. Aperients in excess may affect the baby through the milk.

Retention of urine

This sometimes occurs after difficult delivery, especially if there is pain from perineal stitches, and catheterization is then required.

Breast feeding

See p. 195.

POSTNATAL EXAMINATION

The patient should be examined before discharge from hospital and at 6 weeks after delivery. The latter examination is usually made by the general practitioner. The purpose is to detect any pelvic abnormality that has resulted from the pregnancy or labour, and to folow up such complications as hypertension, urinary tract infection or anaemia. Advice on infant feeding may be required, and every woman should be asked if she needs family planning advice, which can then be arranged.

Apart from the investigation of specific complaints, a vaginal examination is made and a speculum is passed. Even if the woman has had a cervical smear during the pregnancy, this should be repeated unless she has a smear within the 2 years preceding the pregnancy, because antenatal smears are not completely reliable.

Lesions that may be encountered include:

Cervical erosion (p. 249). These should not be treated at the 6th week as many of them resolve. The patient is seen again at the 12th week, and only if the erosion persists and causes discharge is cauterization, cryosurgery or laser treatment given.

Prolapse and *stress incontinence*. Pelvic floor exercises may effect some improvement, but most cases eventually require surgical treatment (pp. 228 and 351).

Uterine retroversion. This does not need treatment (p. 235).

Backache. This is common, but seldom due to pelvic disease. It is more often due to postural defects which are made worse by fatigue.

SECTION B

Obstetric abnormalities

5

Abnormal pregnancy

ABORTION

Abortion is defined as the expulsion of the conceptus before the 28th week of pregnancy. The majority of cases occur during the first 12 weeks, when the entire product of conception is separated by haemorrhage and expelled by painful uterine contractions. In later abortion the mechanism resembles that of labour; after rupture of the membranes, the fetus is expelled by uterine contractions, followed by the placenta.

Causes

1. *Fetal abnormality* is a common cause of early abortion. Chromosomal abnormalities are found in more than a third of these cases.
2. *Maternal immune response*. A recent theory, which it is difficult to set out briefly, suggests that some abortions may be caused by deficient maternal antibody response.

   Trophoblast and maternal lymphocytes share TLX antigens which are linked to other antigens which may attack trophoblast. The mother normally forms blocking antibodies against TLX antigens, and her response also prevents the linked antigens from attacking trophoblast. It is claimed that abortion may be caused by failure of this maternal response, and prevented by injection of donor

lymphocytes, which stimulate the production of maternal blocking antibodies.
3. *Uterine abnormalities*, including congenital malformations, fibromyomata, retroversion (only in cases of incarceration), deep cervical tears or amputation of the cervix.
4. *Maternal illness*, including acute fever, chronic nephritis, diabetes. Syphilis sometimes causes late abortion.
5. *Drugs*. Lead, ergot, quinine, cytotoxic drugs. Purges and oxytocics (except prostaglandins) usually have little effect.
6. *Trauma* has little effect on normal pregnancy, unless the uterine cavity is entered by some instrument.
7. *Hormone deficiency*. An uncertain cause (see p. 17).

Types of abortion

Threatened abortion

Slight bleeding occurs, but soon ceases, and the pregnancy continues. Ultrasonic examination will show an intact gestation sac, and later in pregnancy the fetus can be shown to be alive by detection of its heart movements by ultrasound. The patient is kept at rest in bed until fresh bleeding has ceased.

Inevitable abortion

An abortion is judged to be inevitable when severe bleeding occurs, or slighter loss continues for more than about three weeks; when there is much pain; when the cervix is dilated; or when any part of the uterine contents is expelled. If there is doubt whether abortion is threatened or inevitable ultrasonic examination is helpful. Estimations of levels of chorionic gonadotrophin or of progesterone give inconclusive results.

In a *complete abortion* everything is expelled and bleeding soon stops. In *incomplete abortion* bleeding continues and there is greater risk of infection. In a few cases the embryo dies, but is retained for some time — *missed abortion* (see below). Treatment of inevitable abortion: ergometrine 500 micrograms is injected intramuscularly. Anything passed must be carefully examined, to avoid doubt whether the abortion is complete or incomplete. Surgical evacuation is essential for severe or continued loss, and wise if the abortion is still incomplete after 12 hours. The cervix is gently dilated and the contents of the uterus are evacuated with a suction cannula or with ring forceps under scrupulous asepsis. Blood transfusion may be necessary.

Unless the patient is known to be rhesus negative anti-D gamma-globulin 100 micrograms is injected intramuscularly after any abortion.

Sepsis may follow or accompany any abortion, especially criminal abortion, in which there may also be injuries such as perforation of the uterus. There is pyrexia and foul discharge, and septicaemia, peritonitis, cellulitis or salpingitis may occur. Ampicillin and metronidazole are given while awaiting the bacteriological report on a high vaginal swab. If there is urgent bleeding exploration of the uterus with ring forceps to remove retained chorionic tissue cannot be delayed, but if the bleeding is slight this can be postponed until chemotherapy has had effect.

Bacteraemic shock may be caused by endotoxins liberated by coliform or bacteroides organisms. There is vasoparalysis with pooling of blood in the veins. The systemic blood pressure falls, but the central venous pressure may be normal unless there is also blood loss, and the extremities may be warm. Tissue perfusion is inadequate, and later on the skin becomes cold with cyanosis, and there may be mental confusion. The choice of an antibiotic is difficult and will eventually depend on the bacteria found. Gentamicin and metronidazole may be used.

Missed abortion (carneous mole)

Slow bleeding occurs into the chorio-decidual space, raising hillocks of clot that project under the amnion. The embryo is killed but not expelled at once. There is a history of a few missed periods, but the uterus does not continue to enlarge. Slight bleeding may continue. Pregnancy tests may be weakly positive as long as any chorionic villi survive. The risk of sepsis is small and spontaneous delivery can be awaited. There is a very remote risk of hypofibrinogenaemia (p. 88). An intravenous infusion of oxytocin or prostaglandin vaginal pessaries may be tried, and surgical evacuation is only considered after some weeks.

Repeated abortion

May be due to:

1. Maternal chronic illness; chronic nephritis, syphilis.
2. Uterine malformation or cervical incompetence.
3. Fetal abnormalities.

Apart from these cases the term *recurrent abortion* is applied to cases of repeated abortion with no evident cause. Progesterone deficiency has been assumed to cause poor development of the decidua. Good results have been claimed after the intramuscular injection of chorionic gonadotrophin (hCG) 10 000 units three times a week. However, there is no convincing evidence that this is effective.

Since at least 10% of pregnancies end in abortion for a variety of reasons, out of 1000 women who become pregnant twice, 10 women would be expected to have two successive miscarriages by mere chance, and would probably succeed in a third pregnancy even without treatment. Care must therefore be exercised in studying claims that a particular treatment is effective. Rest in bed, for several weeks if necessary, may be as effective as endocrine treatment.

Obstetrical injury or injudicious dilatation may cause *incompetence of the cervix*. Abortion from this cause usually occurs in the middle trimester of pregnancy, with almost painless dilatation of the cervix, and rupture of the bulging membranes. A torn cervix may be repaired; in other cases a purse-string suture of fascia or silk may be placed in the cervix during early pregnancy.

Legal termination of pregnancy

See p. 347.

HYDATIDIFORM (VESICULAR) MOLE

In this condition abnormal proliferation of the trophoblast covering the chorionic villi occurs, and cystic degeneration occurs in the central stroma of the villi. Fetal blood vessels are scanty, and in most cases no embryo is found. The uterus is full of grape-like vesicles. About 10% of hydatidiform moles become malignant; the trophoblast gives rise to choriocarcinoma (see below). Both moles and choriocarcinomata secrete large amounts of chorionic gonadotrophin, and this causes the formation of multiple theca-lutein cysts in the ovaries. Mole formation is common in Asia and West Africa.

The cells of most moles have the chromosomal complement 46XX, but studies of the banding of the chromosomes and of cell antigens suggest that the chromosomal material is all derived from sperm. Some error in fertilization or cell division has clearly occurred, but its nature is still uncertain.

Clinical features

After a variable period of amenorrhoea (often about 16 weeks) there may be bleeding, sometimes with a watery discharge and occasionally with the escape of vesicles. The uterus is often (but not always) larger than expected, without any of the usual signs of the presence of a fetus. The patient may feel ill, with vomiting, hypertension or proteinuria. Enlarged ovaries may be felt. The ordinary laboratory tests for pregnancy may be strongly positive even when the urine is greatly diluted. The diagnosis is now usually established by ultrasonic examination.

Management

The mole should not be allowed to remain. Spontaneous abortion may occur, or expulsion may be induced with intravenous oxytocin or prostaglandins, but otherwise the mole is evacuated with a suction catheter after dilatation of the cervix. Abdominal hysterotomy is no safer, but if the patient is over 40, or wishes for no more children, hysterectomy, with the mole in situ, may be considered.

Afterwards, regular estimations of the blood level of hCG must be made by radioimmunoassay, for at least 2 years. If the test remains or becomes positive, or if there is uterine bleeding, choriocarcinoma is strongly suspected, providing that another pregnancy, which could be shown by ultrasound, has not occurred.

CHORIOCARCINOMA

This highly malignant tumour may follow hydatidiform mole, or very rarely an abortion or a pregnancy with a fetus. It is an extremely vascular tumour consisting of cells resembling those of chorionic trophoblast. Because it secretes hCG the ovaries may contain theca-lutein cysts. Widespread bloodborne metastases may occur, especially in the lungs.

After removal or delivery of a hydatidiform mole radioimmunoassay of hCG is performed as described above, and if the titre rises or does not fall choriocarcinoma is suspected.

If there is uterine bleeding curettage may show growth, and X-ray examination of the lungs may show metastases. Vaginal metastases appear as purple vascular nodules.

The tumour and metastases will respond to methotrexate, a folic acid antagonist, which is usually combined with other chemotherapeutic drugs such as actinomycin-D or vincristine, given in repeated courses. Chemotherapy may cause agranulocytosis and thrombocytopenia, and alopecia.

ECTOPIC PREGNANCY

The ovum is normally fertilized in the uterine tube. Embedding sometimes occurs in the tube instead of the uterus, and in extremely rare instances in the ovary.

Aetiology

Mild pelvic infection (occasionally tuberculous) may damage the tube without causing complete obstruction, and so impede the onward passage of the ovum. In the recent years there has been an increase in the incidence of pelvic infection, including that caused by *Chlamydia*, and there have been more cases of ectopic pregnancy.

There is also higher incidence of ectopic pregnancy in women who have previously used an intrauterine contraceptive device, presumably because of mild pelvic infection.

However, in many cases of ectopic pregnancy no cause is evident.

Pathology

Tubal pregnancy is commonest in the ampulla, but may occur anywhere in the tube. The zygote burrows through the tubal mucosa into the muscle wall, where its enlargement splits the wall into two laminae. The tube cannot hypertrophy to accommodate the growing embryo and eventually the gestation sac gives way with the following alternative results:

External tubal rupture

The sac ruptures outwards through the wall of the tube.

1. *Intraperitoneal rupture.* Usually rupture occurs into the peritoneal cavity with free bleeding. Haemorrhage may be torrential, or slower when blood collects beside the tube (paratubal haematocoele) or runs down to collect in the recto-vaginal pouch (pelvic haematocoele).
2. *Intraligamentous rupture.* Less commonly rupture occurs into the space between the layers of the broad ligament (intraligamentous haematoma).

In both intraperitoneal and intraligamentous rupture the embryo usually dies, but rarely it retains sufficient attachment to survive as a secondary *abdominal or intraligamentous pregnancy*.

Internal tubal rupture

The sac ruptures into the lumen of the tube. The embryo, together with blood clot, may be retained in the tube (*tubal mole*) or expelled through the abdominal ostium by muscular contractions (*tubal abortion*). In either case blood escapes from the ostium and may collect nearby (peritubal haematocoele) or run down to the rectovaginal pouch (pelvic haematocoele).

In response to the pregnancy hormones the empty uterus enlarges and decidual formation occurs. When the embryo dies the decidua breaks down and uterine bleeding occurs. Laboratory tests for hCG are positive for a time.

Secondary abdominal pregnancy

In very rare cases in which the fetus survives, the placenta becomes attached to bowel or other adjacent structures, which become matted to the gestation sac. Fetal abnormalities are common. At term uterine contractions ('false labour') are followed by fetal death. A retained dead fetus may become calcified (*lithopaedion*), or infection may occur with formation of an abscess containing fetal bones.

Clinical features

These chiefly depend upon the amount and rate of intraperitoneal bleeding. There is:

1. usually amenorrhoea — one or two periods missed, seldom more;
2. always pain;
3. after a few hours, uterine bleeding.

With modern diagnostic aids, such as ultrasound and laparoscopy, early diagnosis is more often possible, even before tubal rupture.

Cases with severe intraperitoneal flooding

There is severe abdominal pain. The patient collapses and may faint or vomit. Air hunger or even death may occur. On examination there is pallor, with a rapid pulse and low blood pressure. The abdomen is tender and distended, and sometimes rigid. There may be shoulder-tip pain. Since the tube has ruptured completely and the blood is still fluid, no swelling is felt on vaginal examination.

Cases with slower bleeding

This is the commonest type of case. One or two periods are missed, then recurrent or persisting attacks of pain occur, with vaginal bleeding. Passage of a decidual cast is rare. The patient is pale and the pulse rate is increased. The temperature is often slightly raised. There is lower abdominal tenderness, and on vaginal examination a very tender swelling is felt in one postero-lateral fornix (tubal mole or a haematocoele).

Pelvic haematocoele

A few cases are first seen with a large haematocoele after several days of abdominal pain. Pallor and slight fever are usual. A large pelvic mass of uneven consistency is found displacing the uterus forwards and the bowel loops upwards. Retention of urine may occur. A pelvic abscess sometimes follows.

Secondary abdominal pregnancy

This is very rare and may be undiagnosed for a time. There is usually a history of abdominal pain in early pregnancy. The fetus is felt unusually easily, and its position is often abnormal on ultrasonic examination. The empty uterus may be felt separately from the gestation sac.

Diagnosis

Cases with severe bleeding are usually obvious. Cases with slower bleeding may be confused with:

1. Uterine abortion. In these cases there is no tubal swelling; bleeding precedes pain and is more profuse.
2. Torsion of an ovarian cyst. There is no evidence of pregnancy and the well-defined tumour is felt.
3. Appendicitis. There is an 'alimentary' history, with fever and right-sided pain.
4. Salpingitis. There is a history of the cause, with vaginal discharge, high fever, bilateral pain and swellings.

If there is doubt, ultrasonic examination may be helpful, but usually examination under anaesthesia and laparoscopy is essential. If a mass is felt beside the uterus the abdomen should be opened.

Treatment

In cases with rapid intraperitoneal bleeding operation is urgent. A ruptured tube is so damaged that it has to be removed. As bleeding often continues or recurs, much delay for resuscitation is unwise; transfuse and operate simultaneously.

In cases with slower bleeding operation is less urgent. An untreated tubal mole or haematocoele may absorb, but without operation diagnosis is often uncertain and there is a risk of further bleeding or infection. In some of these cases the damaged tube may be conserved after removal of a mole.

If a pelvic haematocoele becomes infected it may be drained vaginally, otherwise the abdominal route is better.

For secondary abdominal pregnancy laparotomy is performed to remove the fetus. If the placenta is much attached to structures such as bowel it may be left to absorb. Delay to allow the fetus to mature is unjustifiably hazardous, especially as the fetus may be malformed.

VOMITING DURING PREGNANCY

Vomiting at any stage of pregnancy may be due to intercurrent illness, which a full clinical examination should discover. Pyelonephritis is a common cause, but rarer causes such as intestinal obstruction or a cerebral tumour occasionally occur.

Nausea or occasional vomiting occurs in about a third of normal pregnancies during the first trimester. Although called morning sickness it is not always confined to the early morning. The patient's health is not disturbed and vomiting stops spontaneously at about the 14th week.

Morning sickness may be related to the high levels of chorionic gonadotrophin which are found at this stage of pregnancy. Vomiting is more severe with twins or hydatidiform mole, when high levels of gonadotrophins are found.

In a few cases the vomiting is more frequent and may persist beyond the 14th week, and it may disturb the patient's health (*hyperemesis gravidarum*). This exaggeration of a common symptom sometimes has a psychological cause. It may express a wish to reject the pregnancy, or a need for sympathy. Excessive vomiting of this type nearly always stops when the patient is removed from her home and admitted to hospital, without any other treatment. Ptyalism (excessive salivation) is of a similar nature.

In rare cases the patient becomes seriously ill with dehydration and loss of salt, and ketosis due to starvation. In exceedingly rare instances there is polyneuritis and encephalopathy from deficiency of vitamin B_1.

Management

Simple cases respond to reassurance, sometimes with the help of meclozine tablets 25 mg thrice daily, or promezathime theoclate 25 mg thrice daily. There is no good evidence that these drugs harm the fetus.

Severe cases are admitted to hospital. The few patients who do not improve immediately are given intravenous glucose saline as required to maintain a urinary output of at least 1 litre daily. Oral feeding is resumed as soon as possible. Intramuscular injections of thiamine hydrochloride are sometimes given.

Termination of pregnancy is hardly ever necessary on purely medical grounds. Social and psychological problems may require help.

HYPERTENSION AND PROTEINURIA

Hypertension or proteinuria may be due to pre-existing disease which is discovered or intensified during pregnancy, such as essential hypertension or nephritis. Other rarer causes include aortic coarctation, polycystic kidneys, phaeochromocytoma and lupus erythematosus. However, it is common for hypertension, sometimes with proteinuria, to appear for the first time in late pregnancy in women who neither then nor subsequently show evidence of any of these diseases. For want of a better term this disorder has been described as 'pre-eclampsia', because a few of the cases progress to eclamptic convulsions. The term 'toxaemia' was also formerly used when eclampsia was thought to be caused by a toxin. The non-committal phrase 'pregnancy-induced hypertension' now has some support.

Pregnancy-induced hypertension and eclampsia

Aetiology and pathology

It will be convenient to discuss these after describing the clinical features (p. 80).

Signs

This disease is unusual in that signs precede symptoms. It almost always occurs after the 28th week of pregnancy. The incidence is higher in teenage primigravidae, in women over 35 and in twin pregnancies. It may occur with a hydatidiform mole (when there is no fetus). The signs resolve quickly after delivery, and sometimes during delivery if the fetus dies. The chief signs are:

Hypertension. Any rise of blood pressure of 20 mmHg systolic or 10 mm diastolic above the pressure recorded in early pregnancy is suspicious, e.g. a pressure of 130/80 in a patient with an initial pressure of 110/70 mm. In severe cases the pressure may rise above 200/140 mm.

Fluid retention. Slight oedema of the ankles may occur in normal pregnancy, but severe oedema of the ankles, or oedema of the hands or face, are signs of abnormal fluid retention. A weight gain of more than 1 kg in a week is also suspicious.

Proteinuria occurs in more severe cases, and may be heavy. Blood or casts are not found in the urine. The blood uric acid level may be raised, but the blood urea concentration and renal function tests are usually normal, except in cases of eclampsia. A midstream specimen is always obtained and examined to exclude pyelonephritis.

Symptoms

Symptoms only occur in cases in imminent danger of eclampsia. *Headache and vomiting* may occur when the diastolic pressure is over 100 mm. *Visual disturbances* are caused by retinal oedema, and *epigastric pain* may be caused by hepatic subcapsular haemorrhages. Jaundice may result from hepatic necrosis.

The fetus

Particularly in cases with proteinuria or long-continued hypertension the fetus may be underweight, and it may die in the uterus. Gross placental lesions are rarely found, but there may be spasm or thrombosis of maternal blood vessels supplying the placenta. There is usually fibrin deposition in the intervillous space. Neonatal death may also occur from prematurity.

Eclampsia

The progress of pregnancy-induced hypertension is extremely

variable; most cases are mild but a few progress very rapidly to eclampsia when repeated fits occur, with deep coma between the convulsions. Eclampsia may also occur in the first 24 hours after delivery, but such *postpartum eclampsia* is often mild. With repeated fits death may occur from cerebral haemorrhage, heart failure and pulmonary oedema, liver failure, or anuria due to renal necrosis (p. 163).

Management of pregnancy-induced hypertension

No effective prevention is known, but early detection by antenatal care will prevent dangerous progression. Patients with a persistent or increasing rise of blood pressure, especially if there is oedema, and all those with proteinuria are admitted to hospital for observation. There is no satisfactory treatment. Although termination of the pregnancy is often required to halt the disease, the fetus fortunately is usually viable except in a few cases of early onset.

Rest in bed is believed to increase the uterine blood flow and also to reduce the blood pressure.

Diet. A normal diet with adequate protein is given.

Fluid and salt. There is no good evidence that salt restriction alters the underlying disease process, but in cases with severe oedema the salt intake may be reduced and oral frusemide 80 mg daily may be given. A normal fluid intake is allowed.

Hypotensive and sedative drugs. Many drugs will lower the blood pressure but it is yet to be shown that they improve the fetal prognosis. Drugs such as propranolol and methyl dopa have a limited place for exceptional cases when severe and progressive hypertension occurs before the fetus is large enough to survive delivery. For acute hypertension hydralazine 30 mg intravenously may be used. In severe cases diazepam (Valium) 10 mg every 6 hours may be injected as a sedative and anticonvulsant, but this drug has a severe depressant effect on the fetus. The doses of these drugs are adjusted according to their effects.

The fetus. Except in very mild cases the state of the fetus must be monitored by repeated measurement of fetal growth with ultrasound (p. 25) and observation of the fetal movements and variation in the fetal heart rate (p. 48). Other placental function tests are now less frequently performed.

Termination of the pregnancy is indicated:

1. when the hypertension or proteinuria, although not particularly severe, increases in spite of rest;
2. when the blood pressure is at such a high level that eclampsia is feared, especially if heavy sedation for 24 hours has had no effect;
3. in all cases at or near term;
4. if the fetus is not growing, and especially if there has been an intrauterine death in a previous pregnancy.

In many cases labour can be induced with vaginal prostaglandin (PGE$_2$) pessaries. Alternatively labour can be induced by low rupture of the membranes. If there is no rapid progress a Syntocinon drip may be used. Although there is a risk of increasing the blood pressure the drip is often preferable to Caesarean section. During labour and for a few hours afterwards the blood pressure must be watched, as a further rise may occur and should be controlled with hypotensive and sedative drugs. For primigravidae at 34 weeks or less, and for severe cases at later stages in which labour does not follow induction, Caesarean section is considered.

Treatment of eclampsia

All cases are removed to hospital. It is best if a strong sedative (see below) is given first, and the doctor must travel with the patient to treat any respiratory difficulty which may arise.

Sedatives. Many drugs have been recommended to control the fits. Two alternatives are:

1. Diazepam (Valium) 10 mg is given intravenously and subsequent doses adjusted according to effect. The patient is kept deeply sedated until the fits are controlled.
2. A slow intravenous infusion of chlorpromazine 35 mg, phenergan 50 mg and pethidine 100 mg in 50 ml of 50% dextrose solution; this may be followed by intramuscular injections of half of these doses every three hours.

Hypotensive drugs have been mentioned above.

Diuretics. Intravenous frusemide 60 mg can be given if there is gross oedema.

Nursing care. Any disturbance may precipitate another fit, so the patient is kept in a quiet room. Some manipulations are unavoidable. The patient must be turned from time to time to prevent pulmonary collapse. An indwelling catheter gives accurate knowledge of her urinary output. Blood pressure, pulse rate and fluid balance must be recorded frequently.

During a fit restraint may be needed, and a mouth prop may prevent the tongue being bitten. If the patient is unconscious nothing is given by mouth, and if there is vomiting gastric aspiration is required. A suction machine, laryngoscope and oxygen must be available. Antibiotics are given if she is long unconscious to prevent pulmonary infection.

Delivery. Some patients are already in labour; otherwise, after control of the fits, labour is induced by rupture of the membranes. Caesarean section is recommended if delivery is likely to be difficult or delayed for any reason.

Prognosis

The immediate maternal risk is slight unless eclampsia occurs, but then the mortality may be as high as 5%. The fetal mortality in pre-eclampsia is about 3%, but rises to over 30% in eclampsia.

If a patient has hypertension in one pregnancy she has a 50% chance of it in a subsequent pregnancy, but if she has it in two pregnancies the subsequent incidence rises to over 75%. Such patients with recurrent hypertension probably have essential hypertension (see below) which has been unmasked by the pregnancy. Pregnancy-induced hypertension or eclampsia are not followed by chronic nephritis, and it is not believed that they make essential hypertension worse. The patient who subsequently has hypertension would probably have had it in any case.

Pathology

The morbid anatomy is unknown except in fatal cases of eclampsia; the pathology of non-fatal hypertension is uncertain. In eclampsia the liver shows haemorrhagic necrosis of the peripheral (portal) parts of the lobules. In the kidney swelling of the glomerular endothelium and degeneration of the tubules may be found; renal necrosis is rare. Cerebral haemorrhage may cause death. Pulmonary congestion and signs of heart failure are usual. Widespread intravascular microcoagulation may occur.

Aetiology

The cause of pregnancy-induced hypertension and eclampsia is unknown. The underlying features of both are vasoconstriction and fluid retention. It would take the whole of this book even to list the theories of causation which have been put forward. No theory has so far led to successful prevention. The most fashionable theories at present are:

1. *Altered vascular reaction.* Angiotensin is a potent vasoconstrictor, of which the blood concentration may be slightly

increased in normal pregnancy. Its effect is opposed by prostacyclin, a vasodilator which is present in the walls of blood vessels. In hypertensive pregnancy there may be a reduced concentration of prostacyclin in maternal blood and in uterine, renal and umbilical vessels, with an increase in blood levels of angiotensin. The reason for this is not explained.

2. *Immunological mechanism.* During pregnancy the maternal immune response to fetal trophoblast, which must contain antigens and immunoglobulins of paternal origin, is restrained. Some trophoblast enters the maternal circulation, and if this occurs to an excessive degree abnormal amounts of fetal antigen may be released, and antigen–antibody complexes deposited in renal and placental blood vessels.

3. *Intravascular coagulation.* In eclampsia there is evidence of widespread intravascular coagulation, and it is suggested that this is the cause of the renal, hepatic, cerebral and placental lesions. However, such coagulation has not been observed in cases of mild hypertension.

Essential hypertension in pregnancy

Cases of hypertension which are discovered in early pregnancy, and for which no underlying cause is found, are placed in this category. There is often a family history of hypertension. From experience the obstetrician regards any blood pressure over 130/80 mm with suspicion, although a physician (who is thinking only of cardiac, renal and cerebral disease) would disregard it.

It is found that patients with an initial blood pressure of more than 130/80 mm have a 60% probability of a rise of pressure in late pregnancy, when proteinuria may appear. This is described as 'pregnancy-induced hypertension superimposed on essential hypertension'. The course of events and the management are the same as in pregnancy-induced hypertension, except that the trouble is likely to recur in every successive pregnancy, and that there is likely to be progressive hypertension in later life. In rare cases the hypertension progresses rapidly, but in most cases the immediate maternal prognosis is good.

Some of these patients will already be taking hypotensive drugs before pregnancy; these are usually continued. Otherwise the management is the same as for pregnancy-induced hypertension.

Chronic nephritis

Nephritis is a rare complication of pregnancy; its course is probably unaffected by pregnancy. The diagnosis rests on the history and the discovery of proteinuria, oedema or hypertension in early pregnancy.

Some patients give a past history of acute nephritis. If they only have proteinuria the maternal and fetal prognosis is good, but if the disease has progressed to severe hypertension the maternal prognosis is already bad, and intrauterine fetal death often occurs.

Other cases are of insidious onset. If there is severe oedema and proteinuria the maternal and fetal prognosis is bad, but patients with only slight proteinuria and good renal function tests usually do well during pregnancy.

The management is similar to that of pregnancy-induced hypertension; early termination of pregnancy is only required for severe and progressive cases.

Lupus erythematosus

The maternal and fetal prognosis is bad in pregnancy, particularly in cases with renal involvement, even if steroids are given. Thrombotic complications include placental intervillous thrombosis and (rarely) maternal pulmonary embolism.

Acute pyelonephritis

Aetiology and pathology

The infection is usually due to *E. coli* which enters the bladder from the urethra and multiplies there. If the vesicoureteric sphincter is ineffective infected urine reaches the renal pelvis, causing acute infection which always involves the substance of the kidney. The infection may precede pregnancy, often dating from childhood, but in other cases it first occurs during pregnancy. Routine testing of midstream specimens in the antenatal clinic shows that about 5% of pregnant women have more than 10^5 *E. coli* per ml in the urine in early pregnancy, and about half of these patients with *asymptomatic bacteriuria* will develop acute pyelonephritis later in pregnancy. During pregnancy the ureters and renal pelves become dilated and atonic, partly as a progesterone effect and partly from pressure from the uterus, and urinary stasis occurs.

After acute infection small foci of infection may persist in the kidney and cause bacilluria and also lead to chronic pyelonephritis, with patchy fibrosis and ultimate renal failure or hypertension.

Clinical features

Symptoms most commonly appear after the 20th week. In severe cases there is fever (sometimes high, with rigors), pain in the loin (on the right side more often than on the left) and vomiting. There may be no frequency or pain on micturition, but a midstream specimen contains many pus cells and organisms, and occasionally blood. Anaemia is common. Fetal death may occur in severe cases, and in chronic cases the fetus may be underweight.

Differential diagnosis

Appendicitis. In pyelonephritis pain is usually in the loin and may be bilateral. In a case severe enough to mimic appendicitis the urine will contain many pus cells.

Proteinuria caused by hypertension of pregnancy. In any case of proteinuria midstream urine should be examined for pus cells and bacteria. In pyelonephritis there is no hypertension unless there is long-standing renal damage.

Anaemia. Renal infection should be excluded in any case of anaemia that does not respond to treatment.

Treatment

The patient is put to bed and given a light diet with extra fluid. Ampicillin 500 mg 6-hourly and metronidazole 1 g twice daily, are given. Most cases respond within about five days, but otherwise or if unusual organisms are found, and if sensitivity tests dictate, then other antibiotics are used. Repeated examination of the urine is essential to ensure that the urine is made sterile and remains so. In persistent cases an intravenous pyelogram is performed about 12 weeks after delivery to exclude other renal abnormalities.

Prophylaxis. In antenatal clinics every patient should be examined for bacilluria early in pregnancy. If it is found treatment is given with sulphonamides or the appropriate antibiotic. Repeated courses may be required.

Pregnancy after renal transplantation

This may be mentioned here. The function of the graft is usually adequate. The patient may be taking immunosuppressive drugs, but in practice fetal abnormalities rarely occur. The transplanted kidney is near the pelvic brim, and because of this Caesarean section is sometimes performed.

POLYHYDRAMNIOS

The mechanism controlling the volume of liquor amnii is not

fully understood. The fluid is constantly being secreted and reabsorbed; part of it is swallowed by the fetus and excreted through the placenta. Fetal urine makes a small contribution.

Excessive liquor (polyhydramnios) may be found:

1. In one sac with uniovular twins.
2. With fetal abnormalities. In cases of anencephaly and oesophageal atresia this may be because the fetus does not swallow the fluid, but there may be an excess of fluid with other abnormalities.
3. With rare placental angioma. Fluid exudes from the vessels of the tumour.
4. With maternal diabetes. Fetus and placenta are both large.
5. With hydrops fetalis from haemolytic disease (p. 168). In a few cases hydrops fetalis occurs in the absence of haemolytic disease because of fetal cardiac abnormality.

Often no cause for polyhydramnios is evident.

Clinical features

Acute polyhydramnios is rare, and is usually associated with uniovular twins. It occurs at about 20 weeks and causes painful uterine distension. Abortion usually occurs.

Chronic polyhydramnios is far more common, and is found after the 30th week. There is discomfort and breathlessness, but not pain. The uterus is larger than expected from the duration of gestation. It is difficult to feel or hear the fetus and (in contrast to twin pregnancy) the uterus feels full of fluid rather than of solid fetuses. Ultrasonic examination is essential to exclude twins or fetal abnormalities, although not all abnormalities can thus be detected. If amniocentesis is performed the fluid should be examined for alpha-fetoprotein (see p. 186). The urine is tested for sugar.

There is an increased incidence of pregnancy-induced hypertension. The membranes may rupture or labour may start prematurely. Malpresentations or cord prolapse may occur. The duration of labour is usually normal, but postpartum haemorrhage may be caused by poor uterine retraction. The total fetal mortality is high, from prematurity, abnormalities, diabetes and malpresentations. If the fetus has any difficulty in swallowing after birth an oesophageal tube should be passed to exclude atresia.

Treatment

Rest in bed may relieve discomfort. If there are severe symptoms before the 36th week abdominal paracentesis may be tried. Fluid is taken off slowly through a fine needle. After the 36th week the membranes may be ruptured and an oxytocic drip set up, especially if the fetus is known to be abnormal. There is a slight risk of placental separation if a lot of liquor suddenly escapes.

OLIGOHYDRAMNIOS

The volume of liquor is relatively reduced in late normal pregnancy. Oligohydramnios is also associated with the fetal abnormality of renal agenesis.

PATHOLOGY OF THE PLACENTA

Towards term the trophoblast covering the chorionic villi often shows degenerative changes, and as a result the maternal blood around these villi may clot or deposit fibrin. In addition calcification is common near the decidual plate. The placental reserve is so great that these degenerative changes seldom affect the fetus.

Cysts and tumours (angiomata) of the placenta are rare.

In diabetes and haemolytic disease the placenta is large.

Placental insufficiency may occur in hypertension, renal disease, postmaturity, diabetes, if the mother smokes heavily, and in other cases without explanation. Sometimes intrauterine fetal death occurs in successive pregnancies.

Placental insufficiency during pregnancy may be recognized by:

1. *Failure of fetal growth.* This may be observed clinically, and by repeated ultrasonic measurement of the fetal abdominal circumference, biparietal diameter and femoral length (p. 25).
2. *Observing fetal activity.* The movements of the fetus and its cardiac responses may be observed (p. 48).
3. *Measurement of placental hormones.* Oestriol assay gives an indication of fetoplacental function, but since ultrasound has become generally available oestriol assay is now infrequently used. The formation of oestriol is a complex process. Dehydroepiandrosterone is produced by the fetal adrenal, hydrolysed by the fetal liver, and converted to oestriol in the placenta. The oestriol passes into the maternal blood and is excreted by the maternal kidney. The oestriol output can be measured in the maternal urine. The range of normal variation is wide, and repeated observations are required.

ANTEPARTUM HAEMORRHAGE

Antepartum haemorrhage is defined as bleeding from the placental site after the 28th week of pregnancy and before the birth of the child. It may come from:

1. A normally situated placenta — *abruptio placentae*.
2. A placenta situated wholly or partly on the lower uterine segment — *placenta praevia*.

Vaginal bleeding in late pregnancy may also come from an erosion, polyp or carcinoma of the cervix. Such *incidental bleeding* will cause diagnostic difficulty but is not usually included in the conventional definition.

ABRUPTIO PLACENTAE (ACCIDENTAL HAEMORRHAGE)

Aetiology

Hypertension is found in 30% of the cases, but it is uncertain whether this causes the haemorrhage; in some cases proteinuria and hypertension follow rather than precede the bleeding.

Abruptio placentae occurs most frequently in patients with a poor social and nutritional background, and folic acid deficiency has been found in some of these cases; prophylactic administration of folic acid will not prevent them.

In a small number of cases placental separation is due to trauma such as external version, but in most cases there has been no injury.

Pathology

When retroplacental bleeding occurs there may be a small localized haematoma, or an extensive separation of the placenta which will kill the fetus. A large collection of blood may track down between the membranes and the uterine wall to escape through the cervix (*revealed bleeding*), or it may be retained within the uterus (*concealed bleeding*), and mixed types occur.

With severe concealed haemorrhage blood not only collects behind the placenta but infiltrates into the wall of the uterus, disrupting the muscle fibres and even reaching the peritoneal surface (Couvelaire uterus). In some of these cases disorders of blood coagulation occur (p. 146). Some cases are followed by anuria, probably due to arterial spasm from a utero-renal reflex, which may end with renal necrosis (p. 163).

Concealed haemorrhage

Clinical features

Severe cases are fortunately uncommon, as the patient is severely shocked and may die. She is pale and complains of severe and continuous abdominal pain. The pulse rate may be rapid, but is not always so, even when the patient is obviously very ill. The uterus is tender to the touch, distended and may feel hard. It is difficult to feel the fetus, but in late pregnancy the head is often engaged. The fetus is almost invariably dead and the heart sounds are not heard.

With a small retroplacental haemorrhage the patient complains of pain and there is localized tenderness, but there is little or no shock and the fetal heart sounds may be heard.

An ultrasound scan will show the position of the placenta and the size of any retroplacental clot.

Treatment

In a severe case morphine is injected at once and blood transfusion started. The pulse rate and arterial blood pressure should not be the only indications of the amount of blood needed; measurement of the central venous pressure is the best guide. In cases that respond to treatment labour often starts spontaneously, but if it does not then the membranes are ruptured, and if contractions do not follow a Syntocinon drip is started.

If the patient is still very ill and labour is not in progress a difficult decision has to be made. Caesarean section obviously carries a grave risk, yet if the patient is left she may die undelivered.

In any case postpartum haemorrhage may follow. This may respond to the usual treatment, but if the blood does not clot the treatment discussed on p. 161 is required. Hysterectomy is a desperate measure which is seldom justified.

In slight cases of concealed bleeding the diagnosis is often uncertain. Admission to hospital for observation is essential, and if there is any evidence of fetal distress Caesarean section is performed.

Revealed haemorrhage

Clinical features

In severe cases there is uterine tenderness and the fetal heart sounds are absent; with the bleeding the diagnosis is obvious. In slighter cases in which the only sign is bleeding the differential diagnosis from placenta praevia is often difficult. If the head is engaged placenta of serious degree is excluded. The position of the placenta can be determined by ultrasonic examination. *All cases, however slight, should be admitted to hospital for observation, without pelvic examination.*

Treatment

If there has only been slight loss and the fetal heart sounds are normal no immediate treatment is necessary until the differential diagnosis has been resolved. If placenta praevia can be excluded and no further loss occurs the patient is only kept at rest for a few days.

If the loss is heavy and there is much pain the fetus is usually dead. Blood transfusion is begun. Unless labour is in progress the membranes are ruptured. If contractions do not follow rupture of the membranes an oxytocic drip is set up.

Caesarean section is only recommended for the very unusual case in which bleeding is heavy, labour is not in progress and the fetus is alive.

PLACENTA PRAEVIA

Aetiology and pathology

The reason for low implantation is unknown. It occurs in

about 1 in 200 pregnancies, and the incidence increases slightly with advancing age and parity. A placenta praevia is often thinner and more adherent than a normal placenta.

Placenta praevia may be of severe or slight degree. In the former the placenta covers the internal cervical os (central type). In the latter the placenta is partly inserted on the lower uterine segment but it does not cover the os.

Clinical features

Whenever the uterus contracts strongly enough to stretch the lower uterine segment a low-lying placenta will be partly separated and bleed. This usually (but not always) occurs during pregnancy, but severe bleeding is inevitable during labour.

The bleeding is unrelated to general activity, although it may follow vaginal examination or coitus. It is painless, and often recurs. Dangerous bleeding during labour is followed by the usual signs of shock and anaemia. Unless the maternal blood pressure falls severely the fetal heart sounds are usually present.

Because the placenta occupies the lower uterine segment the fetal head cannot engage, and there may be a malpresentation.

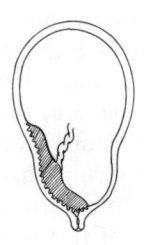

Fig. 5.1 Placenta praevia. The placenta covers the internal os.

Diagnosis

During pregnancy the differential diagnosis includes abruptio placentae, cervical erosion, polyp and carcinoma. It is safe to pass a speculum to inspect the cervix, but unless an erosion is seen to be bleeding its discovery should never be taken to exclude placenta praevia.

Ultrasonic examination will nearly always show the position of the placenta. However, if ultrasonic examination in early pregnancy suggests that the placenta is low-lying, this conclusion is not always reliable at that stage, and it must be confirmed by repeating the examination in late pregnancy.

It is very dangerous to attempt to demonstrate or exclude a placenta praevia by passing a finger through the cervix; this may cause furious bleeding. This should never be done unless the diagnosis is otherwise uncertain, and then only with the patient anaesthetized in the operating theatre with all preparations made for treatment, including blood transfusion and Caesarean section.

Treatment

If bleeding occurs during pregnancy the patient is admitted to hospital. If bleeding is slight she is kept at rest and ultrasonic investigation is made. In nearly every case the position of the placenta is certainly determined. Only if this, and perhaps the fact that the head is engaged, proves that the placenta is not in the lower segment is she allowed to leave. In the very few cases in which the diagnosis is still uncertain the patient is kept at rest until about the 38th week, when a vaginal examination is made in the theatre.

If a placenta praevia is demonstrated, Caesarean section is performed shortly before term. This avoids the haemorrhage which is otherwise inevitable during vaginal delivery.

In a few cases in spite of rest in hospital, or after emergency admission, severe bleeding occurs. The treatment is

Caesarean section as soon as any shock has been treated by blood transfusion. This should still be done even if the fetus is dead.

SPONTANEOUS PREMATURE (PRETERM) LABOUR

This may occur with multiple pregnancy, hydramnios, sometimes if the fetus is abnormal, if the membranes rupture prematurely, and after fetal death. There is a tendency for premature labour to occur if the mother smokes heavily or has urinary tract infection. In many of these cases the fetus is also light-for-dates.

PREMATURE RUPTURE OF THE MEMBRANES

This may occur when the cervix is incompetent (p. 67), in cases of overdistension of the uterus by twins or hydramnios, or without explanation. Strong uterine action usually follows within a few days and the fetus is expelled; its hope of survival depends on its maturity. Sometimes labour does not occur for a few weeks. Liquor continues to escape and there is a risk of bacteria invading the uterus and causing fetal infection. To avoid this risk, if the fetus is large enough to have a good hope of survival (34 weeks) it is best to stimulate uterine contractions with an oxytocic drip. If, however, the fetus is thought to be too small to survive, an attempt may be made to inhibit uterine action.

The myometrium contains both α and β adrenergic receptors, as well as cholinergic receptors. The effect of adrenergic drugs on the uterus is variable, but strong stimulation of β receptors by β-mimetic drugs such as isoxsuprine or Ritodrine may inhibit myometrial activity. Ritodrine is infused at 50 micrograms/minute in a 5% solution of glucose in water, increasing the rate until contractions are inhibited, or a dose rate of 400 micrograms/minute has been reached.

Antibiotics such as ampicillin may be given to prevent infection, but with uncertain benefit. Dexamethasone 4 mg 6-hourly for 2 days may also be given to the mother by intramuscular injection, with the hope of preventing respiratory distress syndrome (p. 192). It should not be given if the mother is hypertensive.

POSTMATURITY

In about 10% of pregnancies labour does not start until the 42nd week or later. The perinatal mortality is increased by about 1%. The fetal head is larger and moulds less easily, and in a few of the cases there is placental insufficiency. Diagnosis is often doubtful. If the dates are uncertain the rate of uterine growth and the date of quickening are rough guides. Ultrasound measurement of the fetal head and the abdominal circumference may help.

Induction of labour is usually advised. However, if the head is not engaged and the cervix is unripe the risk of induction may outweigh the advantage. Labour can be induced with vaginal pessaries of prostaglandin E_2 in a suitable base. Alternatively, the membranes may be ruptured and a Syntocinon drip set up.

A careful watch is kept for any sign of fetal distress during labour. If this occurs in the first stage Caesarean section is required, and in the second stage forceps delivery. Because of this, these patients are safest in hospital.

INTRAUTERINE FETAL DEATH

Fetal death before labour may result from:

1. Placental separation or infarction.
2. Placental insufficiency from any cause, but particularly by hypertension with proteinuria. The risk is increased if the

mother smokes heavily. Postmaturity is an infrequent cause.
3. Diabetes.
4. Obstruction to the cord vessels.
5. Fetal anaemia caused by haemolytic disease.
6. Fetal abnormalities.

Rarely fatal fetal infection occurs from untreated syphilis, rubella, herpes or hepatitis.

The mother notices cessation of fetal movements; uterine growth ceases and the heart sounds cannot be heard.

If a dead fetus is retained it becomes macerated. The skin becomes discoloured and peels, and the tissues and ligaments soften. Overlapping of the skull bones can be seen on radiological examination (*Spalding's sign*), and gas may also be seen in large fetal vessels (*Roberts' sign*).

There is no immediate maternal risk; most patients go into labour spontaneously. Rupture of the membranes is dangerous as bacteria can then invade the uterus. Labour usually follows vaginal insertion of pessaries of PGE_2. If this is ineffective an oxytocin infusion may be tried or the injection of a hypertonic solution of urea through the abdominal wall into the amniotic cavity. There is a very small risk of hypofibrinogenaemia (p. 88), but only 3–4 weeks after fetal death.

PELVIC TUMOURS AND UTERINE ABNORMALITIES COMPLICATING PREGNANCY AND LABOUR

Incarceration of the retroverted uterus

Uterine retroversion is present in 20% of women and it seldom causes trouble in pregnancy. In a few cases the uterus does not rise up into the abdomen at the 12th week and continues to enlarge in the pelvis, causing retention of urine.

The cervix is found to be displaced forwards with the body of the uterus behind it filling the pelvis. The full bladder must not be mistaken for the pregnant uterus. When a catheter is passed the uterus often rises up spontaneously as the bladder empties; if it does not do this it must be pushed up, under anaesthesia if necessary. No treatment is required for retroversion unless retention occurs.

Cervical erosions (p. 249)

These commonly occur during pregnancy. They may cause slight bleeding which can be confused with that due to placenta praevia but they require no treatment. They may also be found at a postnatal examination but seldom require treatment.

Uterine congenital malformations (p. 227)

When pregnancy occurs in a malformed uterus delivery is often uneventful, but the following events sometimes occur:

1. The empty horn of a double uterus forms a pelvic tumour which obstructs labour and makes Caesarean section necessary.
2. If pregnancy occurs in a rudimentary horn this may rupture at about the 16th week, with severe bleeding that requires laparotomy.
3. A vaginal septum may be present and obstruct labour, but this can usually be divided from below.

Fibromyomata (p. 264)

Fibromyomata usually cause no difficulties during pregnancy or labour, but the following complications occasionally occur:

1. Most fibroids grow from the body of the uterus and are drawn up out of the pelvis as the uterus enlarges, but cervical fibroids are not drawn up and will obstruct labour.
2. Retention of urine by a fibroid in the pelvis is rare.
3. Abortion.
4. Malpresentation.
5. A fibroid may undergo acute necrosis (red degeneration), causing pain and fever. The symptoms subside in a few days without treatment.
6. Torsion of the uterus and mass of fibroids is very rare.
7. Infection and sloughing of the fibroid after delivery.

Fibromyomata are felt as bosses on the wall of the uterus. On abdominal or vaginal examination they are not mobile like fetal parts. If the diagnosis is uncertain ultrasound may help. Caesarean section is seldom required except in uncommon cases of obstructed labour. Hysterectomy can be performed at the same time if required, but if myomectomy is proposed it is safer to postpone this until later.

Cervical carcinoma (p. 271)

Antenatal clinics are places where vaginal cytology can be done for women who would not otherwise attend. If the smear shows abnormal cells colposcopy should be performed. If a suspicious lesion is seen on colposcopy or with the naked eye a biopsy should be taken at once, but otherwise the patient is followed carefully, repeating the examination after delivery.

The diagnosis rests on the same observation as in the non-pregnant patient.

Because treatment with caesium or radium cannot be effectively given while the uterus still contains the fetus and placenta, Wertheim's hysterectomy may be chosen for these difficult cases. In early pregnancy the operation is performed without emptying the uterus, but in late pregnancy the fetus can first be delivered by a Caesarean incision.

Ovarian cysts

These may be first discovered during pregnancy, labour or the puerperium. They may:

1. Obstruct labour if they remain in the pelvis.
2. Rupture.
3. Undergo torsion and cause acute abdominal pain and vomiting.

A cyst should be removed without much delay as it may be malignant. Operation can be postponed during the first 12 weeks to avoid the risk of miscarriage, and during the last month of pregnancy if the cyst is not below the presenting part. In all other cases a cyst should be removed at once. If a cyst obstructs labour it can seldom be pushed up out of the pelvis; Caesarean section is usually required to empty the uterus before dealing with the cyst which is impacted in the recto-vaginal pouch.

GENERAL DISORDERS COMPLICATING PREGNANCY

Anaemia

During normal pregnancy the total haemoglobin mass is increased, but water retention causes a relatively greater increase in plasma volume, and a decrease in the blood haemoglobin concentration. Values above 10.5 g per 100 ml can be accepted as normal.

Iron deficiency anaemia

This is common, especially in women who start pregnancy

with poor iron reserves. The fetus and placenta contain 450 mg of iron at term, and blood loss and lactation each account for 200 mg. Diets poor in meat and vegetables often contain inadequate iron, and even good diets may only supply 15 mg daily, of which 2 mg is absorbed. Antenatal patients are usually given supplements of iron, such as ferrous fumarate 300 mg daily (with folic acid 300 micrograms daily).

In iron deficiency anaemia the red cell count, haemoglobin concentration, colour index, mean corpuscular haemoglobin content, and the serum iron concentration are all low. These tests need not all be done immediately, but if there is no response to oral iron in adequate doses (e.g. ferrous fumarate 600 mg daily), and it is certain that the patient is taking the tablets, complete investigation is essential. Other types of anaemia and pyelonephritis must be excluded. Iron can be given intravenously, but dangerous reactions sometimes occur. After a test dose of 1 ml, a slow infusion of iron dextran is given over 8 hours, with the total dose determined from tables relating to the degree of anaemia. If the patient is near term and the haemoglobin concentration is less than 10 g per 100 ml blood transfusion is required.

Megaloblastic anaemia

This is uncommon in Britain. It is due to folic acid deficiency. The red cells may be macrocytic, but examination of peripheral blood is not always conclusive; bone marrow puncture will show megaloblasts. Treatment is with folic acid, 5 mg three times daily.

Haemoglobinopathies

In the fetus most of the haemoglobin (HbF) has different amino-acid sequences in the polypeptide chains of the molecule from those in adult haemoglobin (HbA). HbF is gradually replaced by HbA in the first year after birth, but if the child has some disorder that prevents formation of HbA then HbF persists.

Sickle cell disease occurs in Negroes who inherit abnormal HbS from both parents. Few women survive to the age of child-bearing, but those who do have dangerous crises in pregnancy in which the abnormal cells sludge together to obstruct various parts of the circulation. The fetus may die. Iron is ineffective in the treatment of the anaemia; maternal exchange transfusion may be needed.

With partial (heterozygous) inheritance (sickle cell trait) the blood contains a mixture of HbS, HbA and HbF. Crises hardly ever occur.

Some patients inherit another abnormal haemoglobin, HbC, and if they should inherit HbS as well, crises frequently occur during pregnancy.

Thalassaemia is an inherited abnormality, particularly of people from Mediterranean or Near Eastern countries, in which formation of the haemoglobin side-chains is defective, and the blood contains much HbF. Cases seen in pregnancy are usually of the minor (heterozygous) variety; they may have anaemia and splenomegaly but are seldom dangerously ill.

All antenatal patients coming from countries where these diseases occur should have a blood electrophoresis examination. If termination of pregnancy because of haemoglobinopathy is under consideration, a sample of fetal blood can be obtained by *fetoscopy*. A cannula carrying a fibre optic system is passed into the amniotic cavity through the abdominal wall, and a blood sample can be aspirated from the umbilical vein.

Heart disease

The cardiac output rises during pregnancy to a maximum at

about 28 weeks. This high output continues until term. During labour there is from time to time still greater increase in output. A normal heart easily meets these demands, but a diseased heart may fail.

Causes of heart disease during pregnancy

Rheumatic carditis is becoming less common, but still accounts for most of the cases. In prognosis the precise valvular lesions are less important than the functional capacity of the myocardium. Some cases may be treated surgically during pregnancy, but it is preferable to operate at other times.

Congenital lesions now account for over 10% of cases. Patients with septal defects, pulmonary stenosis, patent ductus and aortic coarctation usually do well. Patients with severe lesions which have not been corrected surgically, and those with cyanosis, seldom become pregnant, but the prognosis is then serious.

Coronary arterial disease is uncommon during pregnancy. Rare cases of *cardiomyopathy* of pregnancy occur, with myocardial failure of unknown cause.

Prognosis

The mortality may reach 5% in patients with heart failure, but it is very low in the others. The prognosis is worse with pulmonary hypertension or congestion, gross cardiac enlargement or fibrillation. Reactivation of recent carditis may occur, or superadded bacterial endocarditis.

Diagnosis

Diagnosis may be difficult as breathlessness and slight oedema of the ankles occur in normal pregnancy. Although soft systolic murmurs may be heard in normal pregnancy, any harsh systolic or any diastolic murmur is significant. Minor alteration in the axis of the heart changes the ECG and radiological appearances slightly, but not enough to cause confusion with serious disease.

Management

If a patient gets through pregnancy without heart failure she is likely to have a safe delivery.

During pregnancy she needs more rest, with help in the house, and often admission to hospital for rest after the 30th week. Adverse factors are anaemia, respiratory infection, and hypertension. Cardiac failure may appear as acute pulmonary oedema, especially in cases of tight mitral stenosis, or as slower congestive failure, especially in patients with large hearts or fibrillation. Digitalis, β-blocking drugs or diuretics may be required.

Patients with valvular prostheses will be on oral anticoagulants. These are continued until shortly before delivery when heparin by injection is substituted.

Patients with valvular disease or congenital lesions may develop bacterial endocarditis, particularly in the puerperium.

Termination is seldom necessary. After the 12th week it is usually safer to continue; cardiac surgery is sometimes an alternative.

Delivery. There is no point in inducing labour before term. Vaginal delivery is best, and Caesarean section is only recommended for other obstetric complications. The second stage of labour is assisted with forceps or vacuum extraction under pudendal block, unless rapid easy progress is being made.

In the puerperium additional rest is given, but there should be free movement to avoid the risk of venous thrombosis. Breast feeding is allowed. Penicillin is given during labour and for a few days afterwards to prevent bacterial endocarditis. At the postnatal examination clear advice should be given about aftercare and family limitation (including sterilization in some cases). Dangers should neither be left unexplained nor exaggerated.

Pulmonary disease

Pulmonary tuberculosis

Active disease is found in less than 0.1% of pregnant women in Britain, and routine radiology of the chest is hardly justified except for immigrants or for cases with clinical suspicion. Neither pregnancy nor labour has any adverse effect on the disease, provided that proper treatment is given. Rare cases of reactivation after delivery are related to increased domestic work and strain.

In active cases the usual chemotherapy is given. Prophylactic chemotherapy may also be given to patients whose disease has been inactive for less than 2 years. In active cases breast feeding is forbidden and the child must be separated from the mother until B.C.G. vaccination has caused Mantoux conversion, usually after 6 weeks.

Other pulmonary diseases

These are treated as in non-pregnant women. For fear of adverse fetal effects adrenal steroids should only be given to asthmatics when other treatment fails.

Glycosuria

Renal glycosuria of pregnancy

During pregnancy the blood flow through the renal glomeruli is increased and more glucose leaves the blood. Normally the tubules reabsorb all this unless the blood sugar level exceeds the renal threshold (10 mmmol/l), but sometimes so much sugar leaves the glomeruli that tubular absorption cannot keep pace, and glucose appears in the urine when the blood sugar level is not raised. This is harmless, but must be distinguished from diabetes by a glucose tolerance curve.

Diabetes

This may first appear or first be discovered during pregnancy. A few women only show abnormal glucose tolerance curves during pregnancy (gestational diabetes). Some patients, including those with a family history, are particularly at risk (potential diabetes), and there may be a preceding history of the birth of abnormally large infants, hydramnios or unexplained stillbirths.

Provided that she is properly supervised the risk to a diabetic woman during pregnancy and labour is small, except in rare cases with retinitis or diabetic glomerulosclerosis. Her insulin requirements usually increase. Control is more difficult, especially in cases with renal glycosuria when sugar is lost in the urine and urine tests do not reflect the blood sugar level. Control may also be difficult if labour is prolonged or anaesthesia is required. After delivery the increased insulin needs fall sharply. The infants are often large (5 kg or more at term) so that labour may be more difficult. Hypertension, pyelonephritis, hydramnios and vaginitis caused by candida are other complications.

Even with modern treatment the perinatal mortality is still about 5%. Intrauterine death may occur during the last month, or if the infant is delivered prematurely to avoid this risk it may die of hyaline membrane disease (p. 192). The incidence of fetal abnormalities is raised, and this is now the chief cause of perinatal death.

The cause of intrauterine death in diabetes is uncertain. With high but fluctuating maternal blood glucose levels the fetal levels will also vary, and the fetal pancreas secretes an excess of insulin, which does not cross the placenta. It has been suggested that this excess of insulin may cause episodes of severe fetal hypoglycaemia.

Management. The fetal results depend chiefly on the degree of success in controlling the diabetes, not only in early pregnancy but in the preceding weeks. Measurement of the amount of glycosylated haemoglobin (HbA_{1c}) in the blood may indicate how effective diabetic control has been during the preceding six weeks. Close co-operation between physician and obstetrician is essential. Patients may be admitted to hospital for stabilization, often from the 30th week onwards. Soluble insulin in divided doses is preferable to less frequent doses of long-acting insulin, and combinations of these may be needed. The fetus should be delivered before the 37th week unless diabetic control is completely satisfactory. An attempt at vaginal delivery by induction is often worthwhile, but Caesarean section is performed if any difficulty arises, or if the patient has had a previous section. In practice about half the patients require section.

The infant may have respiratory distress syndrome, and may show hypoglycaemia, hypocalcaemia and hyperbilirubinaemia. It often requires special care. Lactation often fails.

Acute fevers

In any severe febrile illness abortion or premature labour may occur. Most organisms do not pass the placental barrier, but those of rubella, syphilis, chicken-pox, toxoplasmosis and cytomegalic inclusion disease can infect the fetus. Fetal infection with the virus of poliomyelitis occurs rarely. The treatment of acute fevers during pregnancy is the same as at other times.

Rubella

If the mother has rubella in the first 14 weeks of pregnancy the fetus may be infected, and congenital heart disease, cataract, deafness and mental retardation may result. Clinical diagnosis may be uncertain and investigation of antibody titre against rubella is useful. The titre does not rise until about the time the rash appears. If there is a raised titre soon after exposure to possible infection (and before the rash appears) this indicates previous infection and immunity to the disease. Conversely, a low initial titre and subsequent rise indicates present infection.

The virus may persist in the tissues of the child, and neonatal purpura or hepatomegaly may occur. With certain infection in the first trimester termination of pregnancy is justifiable.

Rubella vaccination of adolescent girls, if universally applied, which at present it is not, should prevent rubella during pregnancy. Women found to be seronegative in the puerperium should be given the vaccine. Those who work in antenatal or neonatal units should also be vaccinated if they are seronegative.

Poliomyelitis

Women appear to be more susceptible to infection during pregnancy, and they should be vaccinated, unless this has already been done.

Malaria

Exacerbations may occur during pregnancy, and pyrimethamine 25 mg weekly should be given in malarious areas.

Toxoplasmosis

This is caused by a protozoon whose sexual cycle is completed in cats. The cats excrete oöcytes which may encyst in man and other species. Infection may only cause a transient maternal illness with lymphadenopathy, but it will cause encephalitis (which may be followed by cerebral calcification) and retinitis in the fetus. Maternal immunity develops, so that subsequent pregnancies are unaffected. The disease is unlikely to be diagnosed during pregnancy, although serological methods are now available.

Cytomegalovirus infection

The virus is a rare cause of fetal encephalitis and mental retardation.

Sexually transmitted disease in relation to the fetus

The diagnosis and treatment of these diseases is described on p. 236.

Gonorrhoea

If gonorrhoea is untreated during pregnancy, infection of the infant's conjunctivae may occur during delivery (p. 206).

Chlamydial infection

This may cause neonatal conjunctivities or (rarely) pneumonia.

Herpes genitalis

If there are active lesions serious fetal infection can occur during delivery, and Caesarean section should be done to prevent this.

Syphilis

Although syphilis is now much less common, every pregnant

woman must have a serological test such as the VDRL test or the treponemal immobilization test. If the fetus is infected late abortion, or preterm delivery of a macerated fetus, may occur, or the infant may be born alive with the disease. Living children may be underweight and show early clinical evidence of syphilis, but in other cases the disease only becomes evident after months or even years. The safest plan is to treat every pregnant woman who has or has had syphilis at any time (p. 238). In treated cases the serological reactions of the infant are tested at 4, 8 and 12 weeks. An initial positive result may only reflect that of the mother, but if the titre does not fall the infant must be treated even if there are no signs of the disease.

Acquired immune deficiency syndrome

This can be transmitted from an infected mother to the fetus, and also to a breast-fed infant.

Acute abdominal complications

Pregnancy may be complicated by any acute abdominal catastrophe, such as appendicitis, cholecystitis or intestinal obstruction, and diagnosis is often difficult. Errors may arise because the symptoms and signs of such complications are attributed to the pregnancy. In differential diagnosis extrauterine pregnancy, abruptio placentae, uterine rupture, red degeneration of a fibroid, torsion of an ovarian cyst and pyelonephritis must be considered.

Acute appendicitis

This is a dangerous complication of pregnancy if it is undiagnosed and perforation occurs. The appendix may be high up and hidden by the uterus. If pyelonephritis is excluded by examination of the urine, and the site of maximum tenderness is separate from the uterus, laparotomy is performed through a lateral incision.

Jaundice in pregnancy

Jaundice during pregnancy is usually due to some intercurrent disease. The commonest cause is ordinary *infective hepatitis*; hepatitis transmitted from infected serum is now rare. The prognosis is good, and hepatic necrosis is a very rare sequel. Fetal involvement is rare.

Any of the numerous other causes of jaundice may complicate pregnancy, but the only ones worth mentioning are *gallstones*, *drugs* (including chlorpromazine and fluothane) and *haemolysis* due to mismatched blood transfusion or infection with haemolytic organisms.

Jaundice very rarely occurs in eclampsis (p. 78). In *obstetric hepatosis* there is mild jaundice with intrahepatic cholestasis which recurs in the last trimester of successive pregnancies, often with pruritus. The prognosis is excellent.

'*Obstetric yellow atrophy*', i.e., fatal fatty degeneration and necrosis, may be a very rare specific disorder of pregnancy, but this is doubtful.

Neurological disorders

Epilepsy

Idiopathic epilepsy may become worse during pregnancy. The patient should continue her usual anti-epileptic drugs. If sodium valproate or carbamazepine are effective they are preferable to phenytoin, as the latter interferes with folic acid metabolism.

110 OBSTETRIC ABNORMALITIES

Chorea gravidarum

This is ordinary rheumatic chorea that has become reactivated by pregnancy.

Multiple sclerosis

This is unaffected by pregnancy, but the additional work of caring for the child may be detrimental, and there may be domestic problems. Termination has often been advised.

Cerebral thrombosis

The incidence is increased in pregnancy and the puerperium. Cerebral haemorrhage may be the cause of death in eclampsia.

Myasthenia gravis

The maternal condition is usually unaltered. Uterine action is normal, but because of weakness of voluntary muscles assistance with forceps or the vacuum extractor may be needed in the second stage. The infant may show transient myasthenia.

Dermatological disorders

Pruritus

Generalized pruritus may occur with obstetric hepatosis (p. 109). Vulval pruritus is secondary to vaginal discharge (p. 245).

Herpes gestationis

A rare skin disorder which recurs in successive pregnancies, with widespread vesicular lesions.

Endocrine disorders

Hyperthyroidism

During pregnancy this can be treated with carbimazole or propyl thiouracil. Care must be taken, as excessive dosage can cause fetal goitre and hypothyroidism. Alternatively subtotal thyroidectomy can be considered, especially for nodular goitre.

Antithyroid drugs cross the placenta, but thyroxine does not.

Addison's disease

This is rarely encountered in pregnancy. Crises may occur, especially during labour. Maintenance treatment with corticosteroids is continued, and additional hydrocortisone may be required during labour.

Phaeochromocytoma

A rare cause of paroxysmal hypertension and tachycardia in pregnancy and labour, which can be very dangerous if the cause is unrecognized. Crises can be controlled with phentolamine, and Caesarean section may be advised.

Pituitary prolactinoma

If the patient has been treated with bromocriptine the tumour has usually decreased in size, and pregnancy can proceed without fear of impairment of the visual fields.

Malignant disease

Most cases of malignant disease are unaffected by pregnancy. Problems arise if treatment such as radiotherapy or chemotherapy, which may affect the fetus, becomes necessary, and termination is sometimes advised. For cervical cancer see p. 271.

Mental disorders

See p. 164.

Various minor complications

Supine hypotension

A few women have hypotension and feel faint in late pregnancy if they lie flat, because the uterus compresses the large veins returning blood to the heart.

Heartburn

This is due to relaxation of the cardiac orifice or to a hiatus hernia. Alkalis give some relief, and sleep may be easier if the patient does not lie flat.

Haemorrhoids

If these are painful an injection of proctocaine beneath them will give temporary relief.

Varicose veins

Varicose veins of the legs may get worse or appear for the first time during pregnancy. They tend to improve, at least partly, after delivery, and surgical treatment or injection are not advised during pregnancy. An elastic stocking is sometimes helpful.

Vulval varices

Varicose veins of the vulva may cause discomfort on standing and occasionally rupture to cause a vulval haematoma during labour. Injection or surgical treatment is not advised as they usually shrink after delivery.

Acroparaesthesia (carpal tunnel syndrome)

Numbness and tingling in the hands during pregnancy may be caused by compression of the median nerve by oedema in the carpal tunnel. Chlorathiazide may be tried, but symptoms often persist until after delivery.

Nocturnal cramps

These are due to spasm of the muscles of the feet or legs, and are probably caused by circulatory changes. There is little to support the suggestion that they are caused by calcium deficiency.

DRUGS WHICH MAY AFFECT THE FETUS

The following drugs are occasionally harmful to the fetus and should only be used during pregnancy if there are good indications and no alternatives:

Long-acting *sulphonamides* interfere with the conjugation of bilirubin, *tetracyclines* may damage teeth, *streptomycin* may cause deafness, and *chloramphenicol* can cause postnatal collapse and hypothermia. *Cotrimoxazole* is a folic acid antagonist.

Aspirin and *indomethacin* may inhibit prostaglandin synthesis and might cause premature closure of the ductus arteriosus. *Phenytoin* can interfere with folic acid metabolism, *ganglion-blocking drugs* may cause neonatal ileus, and *antithyroid drugs* fetal goitre.

Heparin does not cross the placenta, but *oral anticoagulants* do, and may cause placental haemorrhage and fetal bony abnormalities.

Progestogens which have androgenic properties may cause masculinization of a female fetus, and *stilboestrol* may cause vaginal carcinoma many years later (in adolescence).

The following drugs can cause gross malformations and should *never* be given during pregnancy:

Thalidomide, cytotoxic and alkylating drugs, radioisotopes.

If given during late labour *morphine* or *pethidine* will depress the respiratory centre after delivery, but the effect can be counteracted with nalaxone (p. 190). *Diazepam* (Valium) will depress fetal cardiac and other medullary reflexes.

SMOKING AND ADDICTION DURING PREGNANCY

Heavy smoking during pregnancy, especially if there is also hypertension, is associated with fetal growth retardation and increased perinatal mortality.

Severe alcoholism may also be related to growth retardation, and in a few cases to mental retardation and abnormal facial appearance.

In cases of maternal heroin addiction the newborn infant shows withdrawal symptoms, with restlessness and failure to feed.

6

Abnormal labour

DELAY IN LABOUR

Delay during labour may be caused by:

1. Obstruction to delivery by:
   Fetal factors Malposition or malpresentation.
   Congenital malformation.
   Maternal factors Contracted pelvis.
   Pelvic tumours outside the genital tract.
   Abnormalities of the genital tract.
2. Inadequate expulsive forces Weak uterine action and poor voluntary effort.
   Incoordinate uterine action.

Some of these factors will cause insuperable obstruction, but strong uterine action and good voluntary effort can overcome minor mechanical difficulties. On the other hand weak forces may fail to overcome even the normal resistance of the cervix and perineum. In modern obstetric practice poor uterine action is usually augmented by giving an oxytocic infusion.

If the cervix fails to dilate it is usually because the uterine contractions are abnormal or the presenting part cannot descend, not because there is anything wrong with the cervix. Resistance of the pelvic floor is easily overcome by general or local anaesthesia, which relaxes the muscles, or by episiotomy.

MALPOSITION

Occipito-posterior and occipito-transverse position

At the onset of labour the head normally lies in the transverse diameter of the pelvis, or in one oblique diameter with the occiput anterior. The head flexes and descends and then the occiput rotates forwards (p. 42).

In about 15% of cases the head lies in an oblique diameter with the occiput posterior at the onset of labour. In three-quarters of these cases spontaneous delivery occurs by one of two mechanisms:

1. The head flexes well and the occiput descends on to the pelvic floor. It then rotates forwards through three-eighths of a circle to the anterior position and is so delivered.
2. The occiput rotates back into the sacral hollow and then the head is delivered in the persistent occipito-posterior position (with the face applied to the pubis). The larger occipito-frontal diameter must sweep over the perineum (Fig. 6.1).

In about a quarter of cases of occipito-posterior position difficulty arises. If the uterine contractions are not strong and the head remains extended, or if the pelvic cavity is relatively small, spontaneous rotation will fail. If the head remains extended the diameter of engagement is the larger occipito-frontal diameter (Fig. 3.5), and the anterior fontanelle presents. The wide occiput may be held up in the sacral bay and further extension of the head occurs.

In some cases the extended head is held up in the transverse pelvic diameter at the level of the ischial spines (*deep transverse arrest*). This may occur when the head was initially

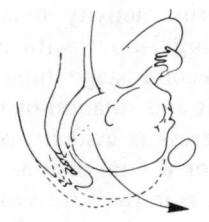

Fig. 6.1 Spontaneous delivery face to pelvis.

transverse, as well as in cases in which it was initially obliquely posterior.

If the head does not flex and descend on to the cervix less reflex stimulation occurs, so that uterine contractions are less efficient and labour is prolonged. The anterior lip of the cervix may also fail to be drawn up and become oedematous.

Diagnosis

The membranes often rupture early in labour. A slow first stage or lack of progress in the second stage should arouse suspicion. Because the back of the fetus is situated more posteriorly the abdomen appears flatter, fetal limbs are felt anteriorly, and the heart sounds are heard well out in the flank. Engagement of the head is delayed because of the wider diameter of the extended head, and the occiput is felt at the same level as the sinciput. On vaginal examination during labour the larger anterior fontanelle presents and lies in front of the posterior fontanelle. If there is any doubt before forceps delivery the hand is passed up higher to ascertain the direction of the ear.

Management

If the first stage is prolonged additional analgesia may be

needed. Adequate uterine activity must be maintained, if necessary by augmenting labour with an oxytocic infusion (p. 47). During the second stage time should be allowed for spontaneous descent and rotation of the head, but if after about an hour no progress is evident, or if the contractions are becoming weaker, or if fetal distress occurs, assistance is required. If the occiput is in the *transverse or obliquely posterior position* an anaesthetic (general or pudendal block) is given and episiotomy is performed. As alternatives:

1. A hand is passed into the vagina and the head is rotated to bring the occiput to the front. The shoulder is pushed round at the same time with the other hand on the abdomen. The head should not be displaced out of the pelvis unless rotation otherwise fails. Delivery is completed with forceps.
2. Rotation and extraction can be performed with Kielland's forceps (p. 176).
3. The vacuum extractor may be applied over the occiput, and with traction descent and rotation may occur (p. 179).

If the occiput is *directly posterior* and is very low it may be delivered with forceps without rotation, but if the occiput is higher or if there is any difficulty then rotation is required before application of the forceps.

MALPRESENTATIONS

Face presentation

Aetiology

This malpresentation is uncommon and occurs in 0.3% of labours. *Primary extension* may occur before labour if, for unknown reasons, the fetus has increased tone in the extensor muscles of the neck. (After delivery the tone gradually becomes normal.) *Secondary extension* may occur during labour if the biparietal diameter is held up in the brim of a flat pelvis.

Diagnosis

This is rarely made before labour. In theory the prominent occiput is felt on the same side as the fetal back (Fig. 6.2). In practice, since the heart sounds may be heard through the front of the thorax in these cases, and on the same side as the limbs, the observer is often confused.

During labour the diagnosis is made on vaginal examination by feeling the facial structures. Late in labour oedema of the face makes this more difficult.

Mechanism

The diameters of engagement of the fully extended head measure the same as those of the fully flexed head (Fig. 3.5).

Mento-anterior position. With the chin anterior spontaneous delivery is to be expected. The head *extends* fully, the chin descends on the pelvic floor and rotates anteriorly and is then born by *flexion* under the subpubic arch (Fig. 6.2).

Mento-posterior position. Spontaneous delivery may occur if the chin descends on to the pelvic floor and then undergoes

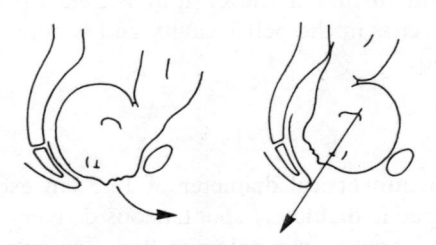

Fig. 6.2 Mento-anterior and mento-posterior position.

long rotation to the front. If rotation fails impaction occurs because the head is already fully extended and therefore cannot be delivered under the subpubic arch (Fig. 6.2).

Management

Vaginal delivery usually occurs; Caesarean section is only required if there is pelvic contraction.

Mento-anterior position. Spontaneous delivery is expected. Forceps can be applied without correcting the position if there is delay.

Mento-posterior position. If spontaneous rotation does not occur after a short time in the second stage an anaesthetic is given, the chin is manually rotated to the front and delivery is completed with forceps.

After delivery the face appears swollen and discoloured, but soon recovers.

Brow presentation

Aetiology

This malpresentation is uncommon, and occurs in 0.2% of labours (Fig. 6.3). The causes are the same as those of face presentation, with one additional type of secondary extension. In this a head in the occipito-posterior position becomes extended still further if the occiput is held up in the sacral bay. This occurs in the pelvic cavity and is only possible with a small head.

Mechanism

Since the mentovertical diameter of 13.3 cm exceeds that of the widest pelvic diameter, spontaneous delivery of a normal-sized head cannot occur unless it flexes or extends. During

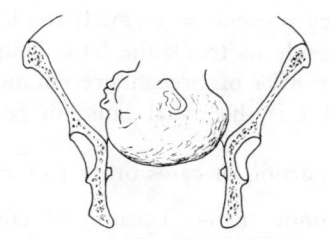

Fig. 6.3 Brow presentation. Mento-vertical diameter exceeds transverse diameter of pelvis.

labour on vaginal examination the supraorbital ridges and the anterior fontanelle are felt.

Management

A head which is extended in early labour will sometimes flex, but if the head remains extended above the brim when labour has been in progress for a time Caesarean section is performed.

Only in the case with a small head extended in the pelvic cavity mentioned above should vaginal delivery be attempted. Manual rotation of the occiput to the front and forceps delivery (or rotation and extraction with Kielland's forceps) is required — this is merely an overextended occipito-posterior presentation.

Breech presentation

Aetiology

Before the 30th week the fetal presentation is a matter of chance. Subsequently the fetus, by its kicking movements, usually adjusts its position to that in which it is best accommodated to the shape of the uterine cavity, so that in 97%

of cases the vertex presents at term. If the legs happen to be fully extended beside its trunk the fetus is unable to alter its position. In over 85% of breech presentations the legs are extended, and this is the usual cause of persistence of this presentation.

In a *small* proportion of cases other factors are concerned:

1. The head cannot engage because of contraction of the pelvis, placenta praevia, a pelvic tumour, the presence of another fetus or hydrocephaly.
2. The fetal position is unstable because of a lax multiparous uterus or hydramnios.
3. The shape of the uterine cavity is abnormal, with a uni- or bicornuate uterus.

Types of breech presentation

The legs may be fully flexed at the hips and extended at the knees (frank breech), or the legs may be fully flexed at both hips and knees (complete breech). The arms are usually flexed before labour, but may become extended during labour (Fig. 6.4).

Diagnosis

On *abdominal examination* the head, which is harder and

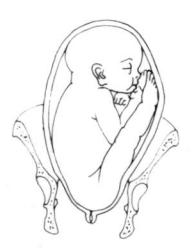

Fig. 6.4 Extended breech presentation.

rounder than the breech, is felt at the fundus, and is often mobile on the neck (ballottement). The fetal heart sounds are heard at a higher level than with a vertex presentation. On *vaginal examination* the coccyx, anus and scrotum can be felt, and with a flexed breech the feet present.

Mechanism

The extended breech engages easily in the pelvis. It descends on to the pelvic floor and the anterior buttock rotates forward so that the bitrochanteric diameter lies antero-posteriorly. Lateral flexion of the trunk now occurs so that the breech passes under the subpubic arch.

The flexed breech engages less readily, and there is some risk of prolapse of the cord as it fits less well into the pelvis.

The arms normally remain flexed while the trunk descends and is delivered. The aftercoming head enters the pelvic brim in the transverse diameter and then undergoes internal rotation, so that the trunk of the fetus (which has already been

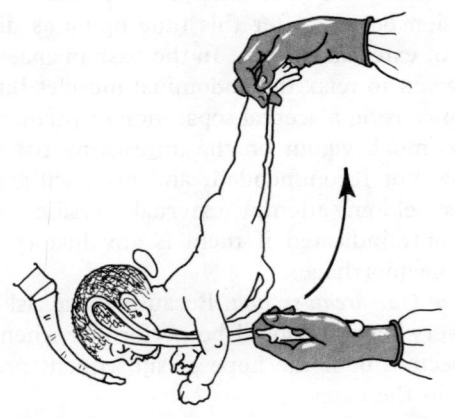

Fig. 6.5 Delivery of aftercoming head.

delivered) now turns with the back uppermost. The face appears at the vulva and the occiput finally sweeps over the perineum (Fig. 6.5).

Breech delivery is more dangerous for the fetus than vertex delivery. The risk in uncomplicated mature cases is about 2%, but in complicated cases (prematurity, twins prolapsed cord, contracted pelvis, etc.) the risk is very much higher. After delivery of the umbilicus, when the cord becomes compressed, delivery of the head must be completed within about 10 minutes; otherwise death from asphyxia would occur. The rapid delivery of the head, or the manipulation required to effect delivery, may cause a tentorial tear (p. 42), or less commonly injury to the cervical vertebrae or limbs.

Management

External version during pregnancy. Correction of the malpresentation by external abdominal manipulation is often possible if the breech can be disengaged from the pelvis. There is little point in this before the 35th week, as in so many cases spontaneous version occurs; after this time opinions differ about the wisdom of external version. In the past an anaesthetic was sometimes given to relax the abdominal muscles but, because of the risk of causing placental separation or premature labour by using too much vigour on the unresisting patient, anaesthesia is now not recommended, and even without it many obstetricians seldom attempt external version. Version is absolutely contraindicated if there is any history or risk of antepartum haemorrhage.

The place of Caesarean section. Because of the risk of vaginal breech delivery section should be performed when any difficulty is expected, or if the hope of subsequent pregnancy is reduced, as in the cases of:

1. Primigravidae over the age of 30.

2. Patients with history of infertility or obstetric disasters.
3. Patients with complications such as placenta praevia or prolapse of the cord.
4. Patients with small or android pelves. The pelvis should be carefully assessed clinically, and with an erect lateral X-ray if necessary, before attempting breech delivery.
5. If the fetus is unusually large, or is judged to weigh less than 1800 g. Its size can be determined with ultrasound.
6. If there is any delay in the first stage of labour.

Vaginal delivery may still be chosen for patients who have none of the problems just listed. In the first stage of labour if the breech is not engaged the patient is kept in bed to minimize the risk of prolapse of the cord. In the second stage the breech usually descends steadily into the pelvis. It will not do so if there is disproportion or poor uterine action, and in either case Caesarean section is performed without delay.

In most cases the breech soon distends the perineum. At this stage a lateral episiotomy is performed under a pudendal block (previously inserted) or local infiltration. If the legs are flexed the feet are easily drawn down. If the legs are extended and there is delay, traction is made in the groin until the popliteal spaces are seen, when the feet can be disengaged. It is not modern practice to pass a hand into the uterus and bring down extended legs.

If the arms remain flexed they will present as the trunk appears; traction should not be made at this stage as it may cause extension of the arms. If this should happen they are brought down by *Løvset's manoeuvre* (Fig. 6.6). The trunk is drawn downwards to bring the posterior shoulder into the hollow of the sacrum. The fetal trunk is then rotated (back uppermost) so that this shoulder becomes anterior, when it will present under the subpubic arch and the arm can be brought down. The trunk is now rotated in the opposite direction (back upwards again) to bring down the second arm.

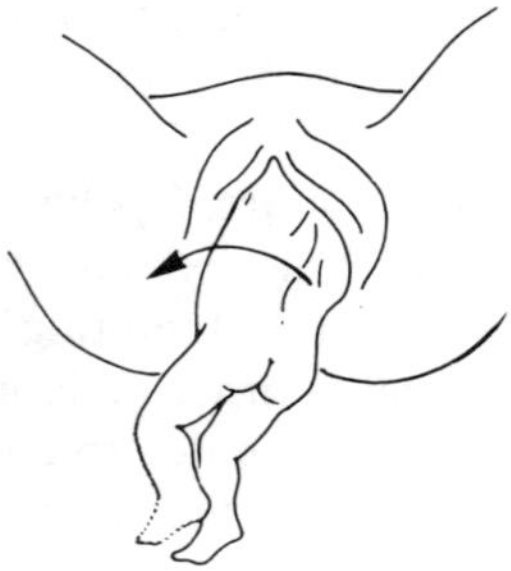

Fig. 6.6 Lovset's manoeuvre

The safest method of delivering the aftercoming head is to apply forceps, holding up the trunk and delivering the head slowly. As soon as the mouth appears the airway is cleared.

An anaesthetist should always be available for breech delivery in case any of these manipulations are needed.

Shoulder presentation

Aetiology

The commonest cause is multiparity, with a relaxed uterus and abdominal muscles. A second twin often lies transversely after delivery of the first. Rarer causes are subseptate (arcuate) malformation of the uterus, contracted pelvis or pelvic tumour.

Diagnosis

This is obvious on abdominal examination. The possibility must not be forgotten during delivery of twins. On vaginal examination a presenting shoulder can be confusing, but the nearby ribs are usually obvious.

Course of labour

With a fetus of normal size obstruction will occur. Very rarely a small or dead fetus is delivered doubled up, but usually the membranes rupture early, the shoulder is driven down and the arm prolapses into the vagina, often with loops of cord (Fig. 6.7). The uterus contracts down on the impacted fetal trunk while is lying transversely. The fetus dies because the placenta is compressed, and eventually uterine rupture occurs.

Management

In multiparae external version is usually easy during pregnancy. The malpresentation tends to recur, when it is termed an *unstable presentation*. These patients should be admitted to hospital from the 38th week so that frequent observation and correction is possible. Near term the presentation is corrected, an oxytocin drip is started, and when the uterus starts to contract well the membranes are ruptured.

In early labour correction by external version is sometimes still possible, but otherwise Caesarean section is best.

In neglected cases with the arm prolapsed it is possible to

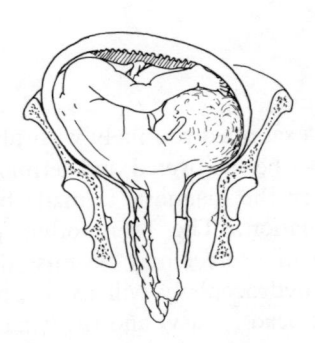

Fig. 6.7 Transverse lie, prolapsed arm and cord.

perform internal version and extract the fetus as a breech, provided that the uterus will relax under an anaesthetic, but if the fetus is alive Caesarean section gives better results. If the uterus is tightly contracted down the fetus is nearly always dead, and internal version is highly dangerous as it may cause uterine rupture. In such a case Caesarean section is hazardous, but is still safer then the alternative of vaginal delivery after division of the fetal neck.

FETAL MALFORMATIONS

Figures for the incidence of congenital abnormalities mean little, as the term is not precisely defined, but it is said that about 2% of infants at birth have significant defects. Anencephaly, hydrocephaly and spina bifida account for a fifth of these cases, and are almost all fatal. If a woman has a child with a defect of the central nervous system in one pregnancy the chance of this occurring in a later pregnancy is increased, perhaps tenfold, but that still gives a 96% probability of the child being normal in this respect. Antenatal diagnosis of neural tube defects may be possible by ultrasound or amniocentesis (p. 186).

The following abnormalities may cause difficulties during labour:

Hydrocephaly

If all patients are examined routinely with ultrasound in early pregnancy this may be discovered and termination considered. Later in pregnancy the diagnosis is made by radiological or ultrasonic examination. The fetus often presents by the breech, and then the defect may be missed until labour. A severe degree of hydrocephaly will cause obstructed labour. Perforation of the head is easy, and the head collapses so that spontaneous delivery may occur; otherwise forceps can be applied to it. If the obstruction is due to the aftercoming head of a breech a metal catheter can be passed up the spinal canal into the skull.

Anencephaly

Early diagnosis may be possible if routine early ultrasonic examination is made. If routine examination of maternal serum shows the presence of alpha-fetoprotein amniocentesis is performed and the liquor is tested for this substance. Ultrasonic examination may be made in a case of hydramnios, or because the presentation is uncertain, and reveal the abnormality. If there is gross hydramnios the membranes are ruptured, and in other cases labour may be induced with prostaglandin vaginal pessaries. Difficulty in the delivery of the shoulders of a large previously undiagnosed anencephalic fetus can be overcome by cleidotomy and the use of a blunt hook in the axilla.

Other rare abnormalities

Other rare abnormalities that may cause obstruction include fetal ascites or tumour, and double monsters, but even with the last it is surprising how often spontaneous delivery occurs; otherwise Caesarean section or embryotomy is used without hesitation.

DISPROPORTION

Difficult labour may be due to disproportion between the size of the fetus and that of the pelvis. The outcome does not depend on the absolute measurements of the pelvis but on the relative size of the head, and good uterine action and moulding of the head will often overcome minor disproportion. Although pelvic abnormality is now uncommon in

130 OBSTETRIC ABNORMALITIES

Britain abnormalities of the shape and size of the pelvis must be described.

Developmental variations in shape

The normal shape of the female pelvis is described as *gynaecoid*. The brim is almost circular except for the projection of the promontory. If the brim is oval antero-posteriorly it is described as *anthropoid*, and if it is transversely oval as *platypelloid*. These variations are of no obstetric significance if the pelvic size is normal.

In about 20% of women the pelvis has masculine characters (*android pelvis*). The brim is triangular in shape, but what is more important is that the subpubic arch is narrow, the ischial spines and side walls are closer together, and the sacrum is straighter than in the normal pelvis. The cavity and outlet of the pelvis are therefore reduced. The outcome of labour depends on the size as well as the shape of the pelvis, and in most cases vaginal delivery occurs, but in an android pelvis rotation of the head from the occipito-posterior or lateral position is more difficult, and the risk of breech delivery is increased.

Developmental variations in size

The pelvis may be small although its shape is normal (small gynaecoid or *generally contracted pelvis*). This is to be expected in small women, and if the fetus is proportionately small all is well. It also occurs in some women of normal stature, and in them the pelvis may be *funnel shaped*, with even more contraction at the outlet. This may be regarded as partial persistence of the condition found in the young child.

Other errors of development

There may be more or less than five sacral segments. The

former (*high assimilation*) is disadvantageous as the pelvic cavity is longer.

The length and angulation of the coccyx vary greatly, but because it is mobile this is not important.

A rare abnormality is failure of development of the ala of the sacrum, so that the sacral bay on that side is reduced (*Naegele pelvis*).

Pelvic deformity due to disease of the bones

Severe *rickets* is now rare in infancy, but it can result in serious flattening of the pelvic brim. The rest of the pelvis is normal.

Gross pelvic deformity any also be caused by *fractures* or *achondroplasia*.

Deformities secondary to disease of the vertebrae or lower limbs

In *spondylolisthesis* the body of the last lumbar vertebra may project over the sacral promontory and obstruct the pelvic inlet. With severe lumbar *kyphoscoliosis*, pelvic deformity occurs.

If there is *paralysis, shortening or amputation of a limb* in childhood the pelvis is often asymmetrical, but normal delivery is usual.

Diagnosis

Before labour

Information about any previous labour is invaluable, including the result to the child and its weight, the duration of labour and the method of delivery.

At the 36th week of pregnancy the pelvis should be assessed by vaginal examination in every patient unless there has been a previous easy delivery of an average-size child. To assess the pelvic outlet and cavity the width of the subpubic arch, the distance between the ischial tuberosities, the distance between the ischial spines, and the curvature of the sacrum are noted. The brim cannot be reached unless the pelvis is severely contracted. If the sacral promontory can be felt its distance from the lower margin of the symphysis is measured with the finger, and subtraction of 1.3 cm from this diagonal conjugate will give the true conjugate (Fig. 3.2).

In primigravidae the head normally engages by the 37th week; in multigravidae the head often remains free until labour starts. In every case the way in which the head fits the brim should be assessed. This is done by pressing the head down, if necessary with the patient sitting or standing up.

If doubt about disproportion remains after clinical examination radiological examination of the pelvis may be advised. From a lateral projection the shape of the sacrum and the position of the head can be determined, and the true conjugate can be measured. Because of the danger of radiation to the fetus other views are not now employed. The outlet can be assessed sufficiently accurately by digital examination.

During labour

If the head does not fit well the membranes may rupture early. Descent of the head may be arrested, but the observer may be deceived as to its true station if there is much moulding and excessive caput formation. If the head does not descend full cervical dilatation will not occur, and delay in dilatation may first draw attention to the abnormality.

Uterine action may become incoordinate; or the contractions may become more frequent and prolonged, ending in fetal death from placental compression and finally in rupture of the uterus.

Management

In cases in which it is judged that vaginal delivery of a living child is unlikely, and in cases in which the previous obstetric history justifies the operation, elective Caesarean section is performed.

In many cases, especially in primigravidae, the degree of disproportion is uncertain. In these cases a *trial labour* is conducted. The patient must be in a fully staffed obstetric unit because operative assistance may be needed at short notice. The spontaneous onset of labour is preferable, but if the pregnancy becomes postmature labour can be induced by insertion of vaginal pessaries of prostaglandin E_2 or by artificial rupture of the membranes. An oxytocic drip must be carefully supervised.

When labour starts a careful watch is kept on progress and for any evidence of fetal distress. In some cases diagnosis of difficulty is only made when a partogram (p. 47) shows that there is delay in labour, and in spite of an oxytocic drip no progress is made.

Adequate relief of pain is essential; epidural anaesthesia is often useful.

There is no fixed duration of the trial; so long as regular progress continues and there is no fetal or maternal distress all is well. If, however, there is no progress during (say) three hours with good contractions after the membranes have ruptured, or if there is fetal distress, then the trial is abandoned. In most cases the cervix will not be fully dilated and lower segment Caesarean section is required.

If the cervix is fully dilated, and examination suggests that forceps delivery is possible, this may be gently attempted under general anaesthesia in the theatre, so that Caesarean section can be performed at once if there is difficulty (*trial of forceps*).

Treatment of cases first discovered in advanced labour

These cases may still be encountered in countries without modern obstetric services. If the fetus is alive lower segment Caesarean section is performed. Dehydration and ketosis must be treated first with intravenous fluids and glucose. Antibiotics are also given.

Even if the fetus is dead, Caesarean section, in spite of the risk of infection, is safer than *craniotomy*, which involves perforation and crushing the fetal head with heavy and dangerous instruments.

In this country *symphysiotomy* (p. 185) is seldom performed, but in countries in which the patient may escape supervision in any subsequent pregnancy a Caesarean scar may be a grave danger, and this operation may have a place.

LABOUR WITH ABNORMALITIES OF THE GENITAL TRACT

Uterine malformations

See p. 221.

Cervical stenosis

After conization or amputation of the cervix stenosis is very rare. The thinned-out cervix may appear as a membrane over the head, when it can be incised; otherwise Caesarean section is required.

Previous colpoperineorrhaphy or repair of fistula

In most cases vaginal delivery is best after a generous episiotomy, but if stress incontinence or a difficult fistula has been cured then Caesarean section is wise.

Fibromyomata

See p. 264.

Ovarian tumours

See p. 282.

ABNORMAL UTERINE ACTION

Each normal uterine contraction starts near the fundus and spreads downwards. The contractions of the thicker upper segment are stronger and persist longer than those of the lower segment, so that the latter becomes stretched and the cervix dilates. Between the contractions the uterine tone is low. At the height of the contraction the blood flow in the placenta is temporarily impeded, but intermittent squeezing of the placental blood spaces may be beneficial rather than harmful. Only if the contractions are unduly prolonged or frequent will the fetus suffer.

There are several patterns of abnormal uterine action. In the past in Britain these were common and dangerous complications of labour. Since oxytocic infusions have been more fully used they have become less hazardous.

Hypotonic uterine inertia

The upper segment does not contract strongly enough to dilate the lower segment and cervix. The pains are weak and infrequent throughout labour. This may occur in a multigravida with a thin and overstretched uterus. Because the pelvic floor is relaxed spontaneous delivery often occurs, but there is a risk of postpartum haemorrhage.

Incoordinate uterine action

This was formerly a common complication of labour,

especially if there was some mechanical difficulty such as an occipito-posterior position or a minor degree of disproportion. The contractions were described as incoordinate because they were irregular in frequency, duration and strength, and the upper uterine segment did not dominate the lower segment, so that cervical dilatation was slow. Many patients became distressed, and it was said that the disorder was caused by fear or emotional factors; but the chief reason for the distress was that the women were in pain for a long time without making any progress.

While incoordinate action may still occur, in modern practice with epidural anaesthesia and oxytocic infusion (see p. 180) most of the patients reach full dilatation and vaginal delivery, perhaps assisted with the forceps or ventouse. However, if the partogram shows no progress after rupturing the membranes and using oxytocin, or if there is any evidence of fetal distress, Caesarean section is performed without hesitation during the first stage of labour.

If labour is prolonged for any cause, dehydration and ketosis can occur, the risk of bacterial invasion is increased, operative delivery may be required, and postpartum haemorrhage is possible. Fetal distress occurs, and even fetal death in neglected cases. Intrauterine infection of a living fetus can occur, or invasion of a dead one by anaerobic organisms.

Prolonged labour should be recognized and treated with an oxytocic infusion, and Caesarean section if necessary, before this dangerous stage is reached. Fetal monitoring is invaluable and epidural anaesthesia often helpful. The urinary output is measured and the urine tested for ketone bodies. Dehydration and ketosis are treated with intravenous glucose saline infusions.

Constriction ring

In extremely rare cases there is a persisting and localized ring of spasm in the uterus (to be distinguished from the retraction ring of Bandl, see p. 35). It may occur around the neck of the fetus and obstruct delivery, or cause retention of the placenta in the third stage (*hour-glass constriction*). It may follow intrauterine manipulations or the use of oxytocic drugs.

If the ring is encountered during attempted vaginal delivery or manual removal of the placenta it may relax with fluothane anaesthesia, or after inhalation of amyl nitrite 0.7 ml.

Cervical dystocia

This term is used when it is thought that obstruction to delivery is due to the cervix itself. If the cervix fails to dilate the usual reason is that uterine action is abnormal, or that something is preventing the presenting part from descending. However, stenosis may rarely follow cervical operations, or occur without evident reason. If the cervix does not dilate Caesarean section is usually required: only if the cervix forms a thin membrane in front of the head is it safe to incise it.

OBSTRUCTED LABOUR

Although this is now rare in Britain, in some developing countries this very dangerous condition is still seen. If obstruction to delivery occurs from one of the causes given on p. 115 the pattern of uterine action alters. Vigorous contractions cause excessive retraction and thickening of the upper uterine segment and abnormal thinning of the lower segment, so that Bandl's retraction ring is accentuated and is so high up that it can be felt abdominally. The pains occur at shorter intervals and each lasts longer, so that they become almost continuous. Placental compression causes fetal death. With maternal exhaustion the pulse rate and temperature rise, and there is often dehydration and ketosis. Particularly in primigravidae there may be a period of incoordinate uterine action or inertia, but this is only a temporary respite. Eventually the uterus becomes tightly moulded over its contents and finally ruptures (p. 185). Before rupture the physical signs depend on the cause of obstruction, but there is usually a very large caput over a fixed presenting part, and the cervix and vagina are oedematous.

Immediate action is required to prevent uterine rupture. A general anaesthetic is given to reduce the force of the contractions, and intravenous glucose solution may be required if there is dehydration and ketosis. If the child is normal and still alive Caesarean section is best, but if the child is dead vaginal delivery is sometimes chosen, although nothing should be done which will increase the risk of uterine rupture. For example, a hydrocephalic head can easily be perforated, but Caesarean section is safer than craniotomy for a normal head impacted above the brim. Internal version is especially dangerous.

MULTIPLE PREGNANCY

Twins occur in about 1 in 80 pregnancies, triplets in 1 in 1000 and quadruplets in 1 in 500 000. There is often a family history of twins. Multiple pregnancy may follow induction of ovulation or *in vitro* fertilization if several ova are implanted.

Uniovular twins arise by division of a single fertilized ovum. The twins are of the same sex and often remarkably alike. If the division is very early there are two placentae and sets of membranes, but usually there is a common placenta and chorion, with two amnions. Incomplete division gives rise to various rare forms of conjoined twins. An excess of liquor in one sac may occur.

Binovular twins are three times as common as uniovular twins. The fetuses are dissimilar and may be of opposite sex. There are two placentae (which may be adjacent but have no vascular anastomosis), two chorions and two amnions.

If one fetus dies early in pregnancy it is retained and compressed in the membranes of the survivor (*fetus papyraceus*).

Diagnosis

The uterus is usually larger than expected from the period of amenorrhoea. Very early diagnosis can be made by ultrasound when two or more gestation sacs are shown. On abdominal palpation two heads and a multiplicity of fetal parts are felt. Sometimes one head is deeply engaged in the pelvis and only felt on vaginal examination. Fetal heart sounds may be heard at widely separated points, and with different rates. Suspicion should be aroused in any case of hydramnios — which is in any case the chief differential diagnosis. The diagnosis of twins can also be proved by ultrasonic or radiological examination of late pregnancy.

Complications of pregnancy

Vomiting may be excessive in early pregnancy and later there is discomfort and breathlessness from overdistension. The incidence of hypertension and of postpartum haemorrhage is greatly increased, and that of anaemia, placenta praevia and abruptio placentae is slightly increased. The usual treatment for any of these complications is given.

Labour may start prematurely, and because of this and the risk of hypertension patients are often admitted to hospital for rest from the 32nd to the 37th week.

Labour with twins

Malpresentations are more common and uterine action may be less efficient than in single pregnancies, and as intervention is often required an anaesthetist should always be available. In most cases the first twin lies longitudinally and is delivered spontaneously. The uterine end of the cord is clamped before it is cut in case the circulation of the second twin communicates. After respiration of the first twin is established the abdomen is palpated, and if the second twin is lying transversely external version is performed, preferably to a breech, and the membranes of the second sac are ruptured. If delivery does not quickly result the second twin is extracted as a breech, or with the forceps or vacuum extractor if the vertex presents. Because of the risk of post-partum haemorrhage the use of intravenous Syntocinon, as described on p. 144, is recommended.

In very rare instances the aftercoming head of a first twin may lock with the forecoming head of a second. If the heads cannot be disengaged and the first twin is dead its neck should be divided and the head pushed up, so that the second twin can be safely delivered.

Fetal prognosis

The perinatal mortality with twins is increased. The average weight of a twin at term is less than that of a singleton; in addition labour may start before term, or labour may have to be induced for some complication. Intrauterine death of one twin may occur, and to the risks of hypertension, antepartum haemorrhage, malpresentations and delay in labour is added that of prolapse of the cord. The fetal prognosis is even worse with triplets and higher multiples, and for these Caesarean section is usual.

PROLAPSE OF THE CORD

This is only likely to occur when the presenting part does not fit the lower uterine segment well because the head is small, or because there is a malpresentation, a twin, or disproportion. With hydramnios or during artificial rupture of the membranes the cord may come down when a rush of liquor escapes.

The prolapsed loop of cord becomes compressed between the presenting part and the cervix or pelvic wall, and fetal death will result. The term *presentation of the cord* is used when the cord lies below the presenting part with intact membranes. It usually escapes a dangerous degree of compression until rupture of the membranes occurs.

Management

If the fetal heart can be heard or the cord is pulsating, treatment is urgent. If labour is in progress and the cervix is fully dilated (or nearly so) immediate delivery with forceps or by breech extraction is effected. If the cervix is not so widely dilated Caesarean section is best. While preparations for the operation are being made the presenting part is pushed up with the fingers in the vagina to relieve the pressure on the cord.

If the fetal heart cannot be heard there is no urgency about delivery, but disproportion or a malpresentation should be excluded.

PROLAPSE OF A HAND

This may occur with shoulder presentations (p. 126).

It may also occur with a cephalic presentation. As soon as the cervix is fully dilated the patient is anaesthetized, the hand is pushed up above the head, and delivery is completed with forceps.

POSTPARTUM HAEMORRHAGE

Bleeding from the birth canal after delivery may be:

1. *Primary*, occurring soon after delivery.
   a. from the placental site
   b. from lacerations.
2. *Secondary*, including all cases occurring more than 24 hours after delivery.

Primary placental haemorrhage

This still is, and should not be, an occasional cause of maternal death. It occurs during the third stage of labour or soon after delivery of the placenta. It is arbitrarily defined as a loss of a more than 500 ml of blood.

Aetiology

1. *Uterine atony*. This heading will include most of the cases. If the uterus does not contract strongly enough the placenta may be partly or completely separated but then the uterine tone may be insufficient to compress the vessels and control the bleeding.

The placenta may also be partly separated by unwise manipulation of the fundus, and then bleeding will occur if the uterus is atonic.

Uterine atony may occur:

a. When the uterus is thin and inert in grand multiparae. Postpartum haemorrhage can recur in successive pregnancies.
b. After long labour from any cause.
c. With deep inhalation anaesthesia.
d. When the uterus has been overdistended with hydramnios or twins. With twins the placenta is also larger than normal.

2. *Abnormal adherence of the placenta*. The chorionic villi may penetrate through the decidua into the muscle so that the placenta is partly or wholly adherent (placenta accreta). Separation is incomplete and the placenta remains in the upper segment, preventing efficient uterine retraction. A cotyledon which is left behind will have the same effect.

3. *Antepartum haemorrhage*. In cases of placenta praevia the lower segment does not retract well to control bleeding from the placental site. In cases of abruptio placentae the damaged uterus may not contract well, and there may also be a coagulation disorder.

4. *Rare uterine causes* of bleeding include inversion (p. 152), hour-glass constriction with retention of the placenta (p. 146), double uterus if the placenta is attached to the septum, and fibromyomata which sometimes interfere with retraction.

5. *Coagulation disorders*. See p. 146.

Diagnosis

This is usually dreadfully obvious. If treatment is delayed or ineffective anaemia and circulatory failure cause pallor, sweating, a rapid pulse and falling blood pressure, and even air hunger. If the uterus is atonic some of the blood is retained within it, and the fundus may rise.

Treatment

Some cases will be prevented by proper management of the third stage. Grand multiparae, patients with twins and those with a history of postpartum haemorrhage should be delivered in hospital.

Immediate treatment will usually stop the bleeding, so that circulatory failure does not develop, and if transfusion is required it can follow the local treatment.

In exceptional cases the doctor is called to a patient who is severely collapsed. The danger is greater if the patient was previously anaemic, or if unsuccessful but painful attempts to express the placenta have been made. If the blood pressure falls the bleeding may almost stop, and such a patient needs resuscitation by immediate blood transfusion *before* any local manipulation. In cases of severe haemorrhage massive transfusion monitored by the central venous pressure may be lifesaving.

Treatment to arrest the bleeding:

A. *If the placenta has separated.* (For signs of separation see p. 53). The fundus is massaged to stimulate a contraction, and ergometrine 500 micrograms is injected intravenously if that has not already been done. The placenta is then expelled from the lower uterine segment by the Brandt-Andrews method (p. 54).

If, after delivery of the placenta and injection of ergometrine, the uterus remains or becomes atonic and bleeding continues *bimanual compression* is performed. A hand is passed into the vagina and shaped into a fist and then placed in front of the uterus. The other hand, acting through the abdominal wall, compresses the uterus against the fist.

B. *If the placenta has not separated* treatment is more difficult and depends on the facilities available:

1. If an anaesthetist and blood transfusion are immediately available, as in hospital, *manual removal* of the placenta under anaesthesia is performed. The fingers are passed up along the cord to the placenta and then directed to its edge. Starting at the edge, and with the other hand on the abdomen as a guide, the placenta is completely separated and when it is completely free it is withdrawn.
2. If facilities are poor, e.g., with a single attendant in a house, it is safer to give an intravenous injection of ergo-

metrine 500 micrograms (or failing that an intramuscular injection of Syntometrine). This will cause a strong contraction which will either separate the placenta, when treatment continues as described under A (above), or will compress the retained placenta and stop the bleeding for a time. In the second event the help of the so-called obstetric 'flying squad' can be summoned from the obstetric unit, and manual removal is performed when an anaesthetist and blood transfusion are available, best of all without removing the patient to hospital, as there is some risk of further bleeding in the ambulance.

If the contractions are still poor after delivery of the placenta bimanual compression is performed as described above.

Primary traumatic haemorrhage

Unnecessary blood loss can occur from a *perineal tear* or *episiotomy* if suturing is long delayed. Any bleeding point should be controlled by pressure or ligature.

With a deep *tear of the cervix or vaginal vault* dangerous bleeding may come from a branch of the uterine artery. If rapid bleeding continues when the placenta is completely delivered and the uterus is tightly contracted this is the likely cause. For suturing a tear a proper anaesthetic is required and the cervix must be exposed with a speculum and drawn down well. While things are being arranged the bleeding can be controlled with manual pressure.

Secondary postpartum haemorrhage

Causes

1. Retained placental tissue. Intermittent bleeding occurs from the time of delivery and may become heavy.

2. Infection and separation of a slough from the cervix, placental site or a Caesarean incision. There may be offensive lochia and fever, and the haemorrhage often occurs after the 10th day.

Treatment

If the bleeding is not heavy and there is infection, local interference is deferred while antibiotics are given. Ultrasonic examination will show retained placental tissue. If the bleeding is heavy, or in any case in which there is a possibility that placental tissue is retained, the uterus is explored under anaesthesia with sponge forceps. Often nothing but blood clot is found and then washing out the uterus with hot saline and an injection of ergometrine are usually effective; packing is undesirable unless bleeding recurs.

RETENTION OF THE PLACENTA WITHOUT HAEMORRHAGE

Retention of the placenta may be caused by abnormal adhesion, or by spasm of the lower uterine segment, which sometimes follows the use of oxytocic drugs in the third stage.

Even if there is no bleeding the placenta should be delivered within the hour. One attempt at expression may be justified, but if that fails manual removal should be performed under anaesthesia. Very rarely indeed a placenta accreta may defy attempted manual removal. It is then best left in place and will eventually separate. Hysterectomy would only be justified if there was severe bleeding.

COAGULATION DISORDERS

Failure of blood coagulation occurs in some cases of abruptio placentae, of amniotic embolism (p. 153) and sometimes when a dead fetus is retained in the uterus for several weeks. Bleeding from wounds or from the uterus may occur. The explanation is often uncertain. Thromboplastin may be released from the damaged placenta and decidua, or from the amniotic fluid. Fibrinogen is used up in forming any large retroplacental clot, and there may also be widespread minute fibrin deposits elsewhere. Secondary fibrinolytic reactions complicate the picture. When intravascular coagulation occurs activators in plasma convert plasminogen to plasmin, which dissolves fibrin. Degradation products from lysis to fibrin themselves interfere with clot formation. There is therefore a complex clinical and haematological picture. There is hypofibrinogenaemia and the platelet count falls. The hypofibrinogenaemia is relatively easily treated. A quick and rough test for deficiency is to mix equal volumes of blood and thrombin solution (50 units per ml). If no clot forms, or the clot disintegrates within 60 seconds, there is considerable deficiency. This is treated by intravenous injection of a double strength solution of dried plasma.

Blockage of pulmonary capillaries by microclots may be more important than bleeding in some cases. For such cases heparin has been given.

OBSTETRICAL INJURIES

Vulval haematoma

A large vulval haematoma may occur during labour from subcutaneous rupture of a blood vessel. This is very painful and may cause shock. It should be incised to turn out the clot and relieve the tension. If the bleeding vessel is found it is tied.

Perineal lacerations

Perineal tears are not always preventable, but attention to the details of delivery of the head and especially the shoulders given on p. 52 will minimize the risk. An episiotomy is always preferable to an irregular laceration, and is nearly always required for malpresentations and operative deliveries.

Degrees

Three degrees are described:

1. The tear only involves the skin of the posterior margin of the vaginal orifice.
2. The perineal body and posterior vaginal wall are also torn.
3. A complete tear extends still farther back to involve the external anal sphincter and (usually) the anal mucosa. If a third degree tear is not carefully repaired the patient is likely to have incontinence of flatus or fluid faeces.

Treatment

All perineal tears should be repaired without delay. Oedema soon makes the repair more difficult. A third degree tear is relatively uncommon, but this is a serious injury and good surgical facilities are required for its repair. For any repair local infiltration with 1 per cent lignocaine should be used, unless the patient is already anaesthetized or has a pudendal block. Chromic catgut or Dexon can be used throughout (plain catgut is too transitory). Non-absorbable sutures are sometimes used for the perineal skin and removed on the fifth day. The points that matter are to make sure that the top of the vaginal tear (which may be very high up) is found and sutured, to avoid tension, and to secure accurate and correct apposition of the various parts. For a complete tear the structures are repaired in the following order: (1) anal mucosa, (2) anal sphincter, (3) vaginal wall, (4) perineal body, (5) perineal skin.

For less severe injuries the first two steps are not required.

After a complete tear the bowels are confined for 4 or 5 days. For less severe injuries no special care of the bowel is required except to wash and dry the perineum after defaecation. A bidet is very convenient for this.

If a perineal tear becomes infected the stitches may have to be removed, and if it breaks down secondary suture is performed when the infection has abated.

Vaginal lacerations

With severe perineal lacerations the vagina is always involved. More serious injuries resulting in *vesico-vaginal or recto-vaginal fistulae* are rare in this country. They may be due to unskilful instrumentation, but are more often due to ischaemic necrosis caused by prolonged pressure from the presenting part in cases of obstructed labour. Sloughing occurs some days later. Rectal injuries may heal spontaneously, but *vesical* injuries practically never do and will require repair some weeks later.

Cervical lacerations

Minor tears are common but unimportant. Deep tears may cause severe bleeding (p. 145) and such a tear may extend up into the lower uterine segment. A large haematoma may form in the broad ligament. This will displace the uterus upwards and to the opposite side, and may be big enough to be felt abdominally. Even large broad-ligament haematomata usually absorb uneventfully, although the patient may be so anaemic that transfusion is required. Drainage is only needed if infection occurs.

Rupture of the uterus

This dangerous accident is now uncommon in this country.

In a *complete rupture* part or the whole of the fetus may be extruded into the peritoneal cavity, into which bleeding occurs. In an *incomplete rupture* the peritoneal coat remains intact, but a large haematoma may form in the broad ligament.

Aetiology

1. *Rupture of a scar.* Classical Caesarean section is now seldom performed; the scar is less secure than that of the lower segment operation and complete rupture may occur during pregnancy or labour.

Lower segment scars seldom rupture during pregnancy but may do so during labour. They are relatively avascular and stretch slowly. The rupture is often incomplete and little bleeding occurs, so that shock is slight.

Scars from myomectomy or from perforation of the uterus at curettage very rarely rupture.

2. *Rupture during obstructed labour.* This is very dangerous, with a mortality of perhaps 25%. It occurs to a patient who is already exhausted and may be infected. The tear is often in the posterior wall and may be extensive and complete. The ragged edges bleed freely and severe shock occurs.

3. *Oxytocic drugs* in excessive doses will cause rupture. In this country, as other causes have become rare, this is now the commonest cause of rupture.

4. *Obstetric operations.* Rupture can occur during such procedures as internal version and craniotomy, which are now rarely performed, and manual removal of the placenta. If the fetus is forcibly pulled through the incompletely dilated cervix that may be torn and the tear may extend up into the lower segment.

5. *Spontaneous rupture* occurs very rarely during labour in grand multiparae.

Clinical features

Rupture of a Caesarean scar is often 'silent' and diagnosis is therefore difficult. With an incomplete rupture symptoms are slight and consist only of lower abdominal pain which continues between contractions, tenderness over the scar (if that is palpable in the abdomen) and sometimes a little vaginal bleeding. Shock only occurs if there is much internal bleeding or if the tear becomes complete. If the scar is adherent to the bladder that may also be torn and haematuria occurs. If there is any doubt laparotomy and repetition of the section is wise.

In cases of rupture during obstructed labour the patient will be severely shocked. She may describe a sudden more severe pain with something giving way. The history of the labour and the situation of the fetus will suggest obstruction. If the fetus is free in the peritoneal cavity it may be felt unusually easily. The fetal heart sounds will be absent. On vaginal examination the presenting part may not now be reached at all.

After vaginal delivery in which rupture is a possibility a careful examination of the lower segment under anaesthesia is made.

Treatment

Shock will demand blood transfusion. At laparotomy the fetus and placenta are removed. *Scar rupture* can usually be sutured after excision of the edges, but if the patient already has children sterilization is also performed. Hysterectomy is an alternative, especially for rupture of a classical scar. *Traumatic ruptures* are often extensive, ragged and infected, and hysterectomy may be unavoidable. Antibiotics are given, and subsequent peritonitis and ileus are to be expected. A *cervical tear* which has extended upwards without reaching the peritoneum may sometimes be treated by packing with gauze.

Acute inversion of the uterus

This rare accident may occur spontaneously, or from pressure on the fundus or traction on the cord wrongly applied when the uterus is not contracting. The fundus, sometimes with the placenta still attached, appears at the vulva or is felt in the vagina, and the uterus cannot be felt in the abdomen. Shock occurs from traction on the appendages which are drawn down into the inverted uterus, and from constriction of the uterus itself by the cervix.

An inverted uterus should immediately be replaced under general anaesthesia. If replacement is delayed shock increases and replacement becomes more difficult. Immediate replacement by vaginal manipulation is usually easy, and 'hydrostatic replacement' with the pressure of water from a douche can has been recommended. With immediate replacement neither fatal shock nor chronic inversion should be seen.

Maternal nerve injuries

Foot-drop due to paralysis of the dorsiflexor muscles with anaesthesia on the outer side of the foot may follow delivery. This may be due to:

1. Pressure on the lumbosacral cord at the pelvic brim during labour.
2. Prolapse of an intervertebral disk during labour.
3. Pressure on the lateral popliteal nerve from a leg support.

The prognosis is good, although recovery may take six months.

SHOCK IN OBSTETRICS

Acute circulatory failure during or soon after labour or abortion may be due to:

1. *Haemorrhage*, ante- or postpartum.
2. *Trauma*. Any misapplied violence during operative delivery or delivery of the placenta will cause shock. More serious shock follows uterine rupture or inversion. Long labour, with dehydration and ketosis, may precede any of these complications.
3. *Anoxia during anaesthesia*.
4. *Undiagnosed cardiac lesions*.
5. *Amniotic embolism* is a very rare cause of sudden shock, dyspnoea and cyanosis during labour. During the height of a contraction a large volume of amniotic fluid enters a vein and death may be due to pulmonary oedema or widespread intravascular clotting. At autopsy the diagnosis is proven by finding amniotic squames or lanugo hairs in the lungs.
6. *Coagulation disorders* (p. 146).
7. *Incompatible blood transfusion*.
8. *Bacteraemic shock* may occur in cases of septic abortion (p. 156) or puerpural infection.

Severe obstetric shock may be followed by pituitary necrosis (p. 163) or renal failure (p. 163).

7

Abnormal puerperium

PUERPERAL PYREXIA

Puerperal pyrexia has been defined as fever of 38°C or more arising *from any cause* within 14 days of labour or miscarriage. The causes include:

1. Genital tract infection (puerperal sepsis).
2. Urinary tract infection (now the commonest cause).
3. Respiratory tract infection.
4. Thrombophlebitis.
5. Mastitis.
6. Any intercurrent illness.

Genital tract infection (puerperal sepsis)

Aetiology and pathology

Organisms enter the tissues through the placental site, or through cervical, vaginal or perineal lacerations. Infection usually occurs at the time of delivery, but may occur before delivery in a long labour, or may occur in the early puerperium. The following organisms may be responsible:

Aerobic haemolytic streptococci. These were the usual cause of the fatal epidemics of childbed fever of the past, but they are sensitive to antibiotics and are now less commonly found in the hospital environment. They are subdivided by serological methods; group A were formerly the most dangerous group, but today infections with group B are more common, and this group may also cause serious infection in the newborn child. Haemolytic streptococci are not found in the vagina before the onset of labour. They originate from another person with infection (puerperal or otherwise) and can survive on dust, blankets, etc., for a time, or can be carried in the throats of patients or attendants who may themselves have no illness.

Virulent haemolytic streptococci multiply in blood, causing haemolysis and breaking down of any clot. If resistance is insufficient there is very little tissue reaction and the organisms spread widely to cause local or general peritonitis, or send showers of small infected particles of clot into the blood stream (septicaemia).

Anaerobic streptococci. The mode of spread of these organisms is uncertain; they are sometimes found in the vagina before labour. They can only gain a foothold in dead tissue or blood clot, which are likely to be present after much local injury. Suppurative foci are formed in the veins, causing spreading thrombophlebitis. The friable and partly liquefied clot breaks down to form comparatively large infected emboli (pyaemia), which cause metastatic abscesses in the lung and elsewhere.

Other streptococci seldom cause serious infection.

Staphylococcus aureus is commonly found in a hospital environment. It originates from some infected person, but survives for a time in dust, etc., and on the skin or in the nasopharynx of healthy carriers, including the noses, skin and umbilical stumps of infants. Fortunately, staphylococci usually only cause localized infection, but septicaemia can be very dangerous if the organisms are resistant to antibiotics, and then multiple metastatic abscesses occur.

Staphylococci also cause mastitis (p. 161) and ophthalmia neonatorum (p. 206).

Coliform bacteria. These organisms are constantly present on the perineum and often cause urinary tract infection, but sometimes also invade the genital tract. They usually cause localized endometrial infection with offensive lochia. They are a rare cause of shock due to liberation of endotoxins into the blood stream (p. 153).

Bacteroides. Organisms of this group occasionally cause puerperal or postabortal infection and endotoxic shock.

Clostridia. These organisms are rare but dangerous causes of uterine infection, more often after abortion than after labour. They come from the bowel and need dead tissue for anaerobic survival. Necrosis of the uterine wall, with peritonitis, septicaemia, severe toxaemia and haemolytic jaundice occurs, with high mortality. The mere discovery of a few clostridia in a mixed culture need cause no alarm — if they are invading they will obviously predominate in the culture.

Investigation of pyrexia after delivery

Every case should be fully investigated and all the causes listed on p. 154 should be considered. The history may help. With genital tract infection the fever usually starts on the 2nd or 3rd day, although severe streptococcal infection may give earlier fever. Genital tract infection is more common after operative delivery or manual removal of the placenta, but normal delivery does not exclude this possibility. Urinary tract infection may occur at any time. Infection of the breast is uncommon before the 5th day.

A full clinical examination is made, including general examination to exclude any intercurrent cause, and examination of the chest, abdomen, breasts, and legs. There are unlikely to be any conclusive symptoms or signs of genital or urinary tract infection at the onset, but the perineum should be examined and a pelvic examination made. In every case bacteriological investigation is required:

ABNORMAL PUERPERIUM 157

1. A high vaginal swab is taken for both aerobic and anaerobic bacterial culture, and all organisms are tested for sensitivity to antibiotics.
2. A midstream specimen of urine or one obtained by suprapubic bladder puncture is examined bacteriologically.
3. If there is high or recurrent fever a blood culture is made.

Clinical events

The following types of cases can be distinguished, although they obviously overlap to some extent:

1. Localized infection.
    a. *Perineal infection.* If the sutures are removed resolution usually occurs rapidly, and further spread is rare.
    b. *Endometritis.* Often there are no symptoms or signs except fever of about 38.5°C. Sometimes the lochia is offensive (but not in streptococcal cases) and uterine involution may be delayed. Most cases resolve in a few days even without treatment, but with antibiotics resolution often occurs in 48 hours.
2. Spread to structures around the uterus.
    The time when this occurs depends on the virulence of the organisms, but it is often after the 4th day. The fever and tachycardia of the initial endometritis increase, and there is lower abdominal pain. At this stage both the pelvic peritoneum and the loose cellular tissue at the side of the cervix and vagina (sometimes called the parametrium) become inflamed. Because of the *pelvic peritonitis* there is lower abdominal tenderness, and vaginal examination causes pain. The peritonitis usually resolves, but sometimes an abscess forms which may point into the rectum or above the inguinal ligament.

    Pelvic cellulitis (parametritis) also usually resolves, but sometimes takes several weeks to do so. An inflammatory induration is found on one or both sides of the cervix, fixing it firmly.

Especially with anaerobic streptococcal infections widespread *thrombophlebitis* of the pelvic veins may occur, sometimes spreading downwards to the femoral vein or upwards to the iliac veins. There is a swollen 'white leg', and also infected emboli may be thrown off to cause repeated pyrexial episodes and metastatic lung abscesses.

The infection may involve the uterine tubes, causing *salpingitis* and infertility.

3. Generalized peritonitis.

   When haemolytic streptococcal infections were prevalent and antibiotics were not available, spread to the general peritoneal cavity was disastrous, giving a mortality of 75%. The pulse rate rose rapidly to 140 or more per minute, with fever of variable degree. Abdominal distention with little pain or guarding often occurred.

4. Septicaemia.

   This was also disastrous in the past but most organisms now respond well to antibiotics. The temperature is very high, swinging up to peaks of 40.5°C with rigors. Also see bacteraemic shock, p. 156.

Prevention

Anyone with a streptococcal or staphylococcal lesion (e.g. a sore throat or a paronychia) should not attend on labouring or lying-in-women. Any patient with a puerperal or other significant infection must be isolated.

Sterilized gloves must be worn for any pelvic examination. Proper care during vaginal examination is important, and such examinations should not be made unnecessarily. Catheterization is avoided whenever possible. If a midstream specimen is not satisfactory, suprapubic bladder puncture gives a better specimen for bacteriological purposes than catheterization.

Treatment

The immediate use of an appropriate antibiotic will prevent most of the events described above. If there is serious fear of a genital tract infection (e.g. with fever after criminal abortion or after long labour) treatment with ampicillin and metronidazole may be started at once, and modified if necessary when the bacteriological report is available.

The uterus should only be explored if bleeding and ultrasonic examination suggest that placental tissue is retained. Occasionally surgical treatment is required for a pelvic or metastatic abscess.

For the rare clostridial infections antiserum is required as well as penicillin, and these are the only cases in which the desperate measure of hysterectomy might be seriously considered. Hyperbaric oxygen may be used.

Infection of the urinary tract

This is common in the early puerperium, either as a recurrence of an infection which was present during pregnancy, or as a result of catherization and trauma to the bladder during labour. *E. coli* is the commonest organism found, but *Strep. faecalis*, *B. proteus* or mixed infections may be discovered. The genital tract may be invaded at the same time.

Often the only clinical sign is mild fever, and there may be no urinary symptoms. The infection is usually confined to the lower urinary tract, but acute pyelonephritis occasionally occurs. Diagnosis rests on microscopical and bacteriological examination of a midstream or suprapubic specimen of urine.

Treatment will depend on the organisms found, and their

sensitivity, but most cases respond to ampicillin 500 mg 6-hourly.

ABNORMALITIES OF THE BREAST

Acute engorgement

On about the 4th day the breasts may become tense and painful because of hyperaemia and the onset of secretion of milk into the acini. The tension within the fascial compartments interferes with the outflow of milk, which is the natural method of relief. Slight pyrexia may occur, but other possible causes of fever must be excluded. The breasts should be well supported. Manual expression or the use of an electric pump may be tried, but are often too painful.

Inhibition of lactation

Lactation can be suppressed with bromocriptine, 2.5 mg orally twice daily for 14 days. It inhibits the pituitary secretion of prolactin.

Cracked nipples

Small fissures may occur on the nipple or areola if the infant chews too vigorously or for too long when there is insufficient milk. Cracks are acutely painful, and sometimes bleed, so that the infant may swallow and then vomit blood.

Treatment. Cracks should be prevented by careful supervision of the early feeds. The only effective treatment is to stop feeding from that breast for 24 to 48 hours, and to express the milk. Any local antiseptic application should not poison the baby, stick to the fissure or cause skin sensitization. Flavine in paraffin is recommended. If the fissure does not heal in this time breast feeding usually has to be abandoned.

ABNORMAL PUERPERIUM

Acute mastitis

This is due to invasion of the ducts by *Staphylococcus aureus*, which may be carried by healthy attendants or babies. Epidemics may occur in hospital. Organisms may also enter the superficial tissues through a cracked nipple, but this is not the usual entry.

Clinical features. Mastitis may occur at any time after the 4th day of the puerperium. Fever (40°C) and pain occur. A sector of the breast is hyperaemic, tense and tender. Axillary glands may be enlarged. If suppuration occurs a localized abscess may form and point, or spreading infection may cause widespread disorganization of the breast.

Treatment. The milk is cultured, and while the report on the sensitivity of the organisms is awaited antibiotic treatment may be started. In hospital staphylococci may be penicillin resistant, but the characteristics of the prevalent strain are often known. The breast is supported, feeding is stopped from that side, and the milk is expressed. If the skin shows brawny oedema, even without fluctuation, pus is likely to be present and an incision is made.

Galactocoele

A small painless cyst may occur on one of the ducts near the areola. If it persists it is excised.

Carcinoma of the lactating breast

This is rare but lethal. Florid encephaloid cancer during lactation must not be mistaken for a breast abscess.

VENOUS THROMBOSIS

Thrombosis of superficial veins in the legs

This may occur after delivery, especially if the veins are

varicose. A tender segment is felt. Pulmonary embolism rarely follows, so that anticoagulants are not used and ambulation is encouraged. Varicose veins may need subsequent surgical treatment.

Thrombosis of deep veins in the legs

This may occur after delivery (and, rarely, during pregnancy), without any evidence of infection. It is commoner after Caesarean section than after vaginal delivery. The calf veins are usually first involved. Venograms show that thrombosis of these veins may occur without symptoms, but there may be pain, swelling in the leg, pain on dorsiflexion of the foot, and a slight rise of temperature and pulse rate, usually noticed before the 7th day. In a few severe cases with spreading thrombosis and superadded vascular spasm the limb is white or blue. There are two dangers:

1. *Pulmonary embolism.* The risk of this complication is about 12 times greater after Caesarean section than after vaginal delivery. It often occurs without any previous complaint of pain or swelling in the legs. Any patient who has previously had deep vein thrombosis or a pulmonary embolus should be given anticoagulant treatment (in the form of subcutaneous heparin injections) throughout the antenatal period.
2. Permanent impairment of the circulation in the leg.

Treatment. Early ambulation after delivery reduces the risk of deep thrombosis. If it occurs anticoagulant drugs will certainly increase the rate of recovery of the limb, and may reduce the risk of embolism. Intravenous administration of heparin is started at once (10 000 units 8-hourly for 48 hours), and an oral anticoagulant such as warfarin sodium. An initial dose of 50 mg is given; the prothrombin time is measured and subsequent doses of oral anticoagulant (usually between 3 and 10 mg daily in divided doses) are adjusted to increase this two- or threefold.

The leg should be rested for 2 or 3 days until the pain is less and the anticoagulants have begun their work, and then activity should gradually be restored. An elastic stocking may be used for a time.

Thrombosis of pelvic veins

Thrombosis of pelvic veins may be caused by infection.

POSTPARTUM PITUITARY NECROSIS

This is a rare sequel of severe and prolonged shock, usually caused by postpartum haemorrhage. Thrombosis of the vessels supplying the anterior lobe of the pituitary gland causes ischaemic necrosis. There is deficiency of prolactin and of gonadotrophic, corticotrophic and thyrotrophic hormones. Failure of lactation is followed by genital atrophy, loss of pubic hair, and amenorrhoea. The patient is lethargic, with anorexia, hypotension and hypoglycaemia, and a low basal metabolic rate. She usually gains weight. Treatment with cortisone, thyroxine and norethandrolone (an anabolic steroid) may cause some improvement. If the patient is not severely ill and wishes for another pregnancy, induction of ovulation with hMG may be tried (p. 325).

RENAL CORTICAL NECROSIS AND LOWER NEPHRON NECROSIS

These rare conditions, which may follow abruptio placentae or septic abortion, cause anuria after delivery. To circulatory failure and anaemia is added the effect of reflex spasm of the renal arterioles. In cases of bilateral renal cortical necrosis all the glomeruli and parts of all the tubules are killed by ischaemia. In lower nephron necrosis there is widespread damage to tubules, but many will recover.

In both cases anuria occurs, with a progressive rise in the blood urea concentration. If the case is one of cortical necrosis death is inevitable unless renal dialysis is performed. In tubular necrosis spontaneous diuresis and recovery may occur after about 10 days.

Treatment. Glucose saline solution is given intravenously, but the fluid intake must not exceed the loss by perspiration and sweating. If diuresis does not occur in a few days dialysis by the artificial kidney is required and possibly eventual renal transplantation.

MENTAL ILLNESS

During pregnancy and the puerperium women have to make adjustments to many new emotional experiences. Most women are ambivalent in their reactions. The wish for pregnancy and the desire to have children (whether determined by innate character or by imitation of other women) are counterbalanced by anxieties about labour, the unborn child, relations with her husband, and many practical domestic and economic problems. Minor symptoms, such as vomiting or insomnia, may be a reflection of these feelings. Kindness, understanding and wise counsel from doctors, midwives and relatives will assist in the adjustment, which most women make admirably.

Immediate contact of mother and baby after delivery, and breast feeding, may increase 'bonding', whereas separation during the early weeks because of illness of one or the other may have an adverse effect. If bonding does not occur, or if there are social problems, the risk of 'baby battering' or of maladjustment is increased.

Significant psychological illness occurs in a few patients.

Most of these have pre-existing instability and would react badly to any stress; pregnancy is not the specific cause of their mental illness.

Persistent insomnia, confusion, any obsession or hallucination, or any threat to the baby should be taken seriously, and expert advice sought. *Depression* may occur in early pregnancy, and is common as a transient attack of 'fifth-day blues' in the early puerperium. More severe depression can be a serious puerperal illness with a real danger of suicide or infanticide. *Acute mania* is rare. *Schizophrenia* may recur or first appear after delivery. Prolonged puerperal fever used to be followed by toxic '*confusional insanity*', but this is now rare.

Treatment of these conditions falls to the psychiatrist, but problems arise with the family and the care of the baby. Special mother-and-baby units can be very helpful. Fortunately the prognosis is usually good, and certification is seldom required.

Termination of pregnancy

Firm psychiatric indications for termination only arise if the psychiatrist is unable to treat the patient by any other method, if spontaneous recovery is unlikely, or if any threat of suicide is real, but these indications are very often justifiably extended because of grave social problems. Sterilization may need consideration.

8

The fetus at risk in late pregnancy and during labour

Apart from mechanical problems during labour caused by malpresentations and disproportion, which may often be anticipated by antenatal care, some other cases of high fetal risk are foreseeable, and women with any of them should be cared for in fully equipped units with experienced staff.

Perinatal mortality increases when *maternal age* exceeds about 30 years, chiefly because of the more frequent need for operative delivery, and the increased incidence of hypertension and congenital malformations. The risk is also increased in women of *social classes IV and V*, because of poor nutrition and physique, premature labour and high parity, and sometimes because of lack of regular obstetric care.

Placental function may be impaired with *pregnancy-induced hypertension* or essential hypertension, or (uncommonly) nephritis. With *urinary tract infection* the fetus is unlikely to die, but it may be both small-for-dates and born early. If the fetus survives an acute episode of *antepartum haemorrhage* the placenta may be left damaged. With *multiple pregnancies* one or more of the fetuses may be small because of placental inadequacy. In some cases of *postmaturity* placental insufficiency occurs.

If the mother *smokes heavily* the fetus tends to be small, especially if there is also hypertension. The reason is uncertain; it is more likely to be vascular spasm in the placental vessels than an increased blood level of carbon monoxide, although the latter occurs.

Haemolytic disease and *diabetes* are other conditions of fetal risk that can be recognized during pregnancy.

In the absence of placental insufficiency, if the fetus is born prematurely, whether spontaneously or by induction, it will be small; but only to the degree expected from the gestational age, and death before or during labour is uncommon. With placental insufficiency, however, the fetus tends to be light-for-dates and may die *in utero*.

During pregnancy warning of high fetal risk may be derived from the obstetric history, or by observing that the fetus is not growing normally, with the help of ultrasonic measurements. It may then be monitored during pregnancy by observing whether it shows normal responses in its movements and heart rate (p. 48).

If the fetus is thought to be at risk the patient must be delivered in a fully equipped obstetric unit, and when neonatal difficulties are anticipated she should be delivered in a unit with a full paediatric special-care facilities.

With all these conditions there is an increased incidence of fetal distress during labour, and to clinical vigilance it is desirable to add electronic monitoring of the fetal heart rate, with fetal blood sampling when appropriate (see p. 48).

If fetal distress occurs during the first stage of labour Caesearean section is indicated, and in the second stage forceps delivery.

9

Haemolytic disease

During pregnancy, and especially during labour, a few fetal blood cells may enter the maternal circulation. The fetus may inherit from its father red cells bearing antigens that differ from those of the mother, and to which she may produce antibodies that cross the placenta and cause haemolysis of fetal red cells.

Fetal red cells may also enter the maternal circulation during spontaneous or induced abortion, and incompatible cells may be introduced by mismatched blood transfusion.

Effect on the fetus or newborn child

If the fetus is severely affected it becomes anaemic, and cardiac failure eventually causes generalized oedema, ascites and pleural effusions (*hydrops fetalis*). Intrauterine death almost invariably occurs, between the 28th week and term. The placenta is large and oedematous, and all the primitive centres of red cell formation (liver, spleen, lymph glands) remain active (*erythroblastosis fetalis*). The fetus, placenta and liquor amnii are bile-stained.

In moderately severe cases the fetus is born alive, but deep jaundice soon appears (*icterus gravis neonatorum*). While the fetus is in the uterus the placenta removes much of the excess bilirubin produced by destruction of red cells, but after birth haemolysis continues for a time and the liver is unable to conjugate all the bilirubin. The liver may be enlarged. High levels of bilirubin in the blood (over 340 mmol/l) damage the basal nuclei of the brain (*kernicterus*). Neck rigidity, nystagmus and twitching occur, and if the child survives there is spasticity or mental retardation.

In mild cases *haemolytic anaemia* occurs in the first fortnight, but jaundice is slight. Nucleated red cells may be found in the blood.

Rhesus antigens

Until recently most cases of haemolytic disease were caused by rhesus incompatibility, but now that effective prophylaxis against this is available cases caused by other antigens are more often encountered. The red cells of 85% of Caucasians carry the rhesus D factor, which is inherited as a Mendelian dominant. If the father is homozygous for this factor all his children will have the D factor (rhesus positive). If he is heterozygous half his children will have it, while the others will have the d factor (rhesus negative). In Britain the calculated incidence of rhesus incompatibilty is about 8% of pregnancies, but in fact the fetus is involved in only 0.5% of cases because the volume of fetal blood transfused and the maternal response to the antigen is variable, and because any fetal cells which are ABO incompatible are agglutinated and may not induce rhesus immunity reaction.

The risk of feto-maternal transfusion is slight during normal pregnancy, and rhesus haemolytic disease is therefore uncommon during a first pregnancy. However, at the first delivery a large number of fetal cells may enter the maternal circulation and cause sensitization, and in any subsequent pregnancy even a small number of fetal cells that carry the appropriate antigen will evoke large amounts of antibody. The antibody is detected in the maternal blood during pregnancy.

ABO incompatibilty

If the fetus has an A or B blood group which is not possessed by the mother haemolytic disease might be expected to occur, but in fact it is uncommon. Natural antibodies to A or B antigens have IgM molecular size and do not cross the placenta, but smaller IgG antibodies may be found in group O mothers, and these will cross. A and B substances occur widely in fetal tissues, so that most of the antibodies may be absorbed by cells other than red blood cells.

A few cases of A or B haemolytic disease occur, but are often mild and may not need exchange transfusion. However, they may occur in first pregnancies. The mother's blood will contain a rising titre of A or B agglutinins.

Other antigens

Haemolytic disease may occur with Kell antigens, rhesus e antigens and other rare antigens.

Diagnosis

All antenatal patients must have their blood group determined, and those that are rhesus negative are also tested for Rh antibodies, both early in pregnancy and at the 30th and 36th weeks. Those with antibodies need more frequent tests. High or rising levels are danger signals. Amniocentesis may be necessary to assess the degree of fetal risk (see below).

Ideally, tests to exclude A, B, Kell and other antibodies should be performed as a routine. However, many of these cases are mild, and will only require treatment after delivery.

The history of previous pregnancies may be helpful, and sometimes the husband's blood is also examined to determine his genetic pattern.

After delivery the child's blood group is determined and

HAEMOLYTIC DISEASE

Coombs' test is performed. This is a non-specific test to show whether the red cells are coated with antibody. It is not helpful in cases of A or B sensitization. The haemoglobin level is repeatedly estimated. Reticulocytosis is often seen.

Prevention of rhesus sensitization

If an injection of anti-D globulin (100 micrograms intramuscularly) is given to a rhesus negative mother (who has not been sensitized previously) within 48 hours of the birth of a rhesus positive baby most cases of rhesus sensitization can be prevented. The globulin is obtained from the blood of another patient or volunteer who has been immunized. The number of fetal cells in the maternal blood after delivery can be roughly estimated by the Kleihauer method of staining a film, which distinguishes cells with fetal haemoglobin. The risk of sensitization is greater if the fetal cell count is high, and also if the fetal and maternal cells are ABO compatible. The globulin blocks the immunity reaction to D cells, but the mechanism is still uncertain; it is probably not due to simple elimination of D cells from the blood.

Treatment

The assessment of severity of haemolytic disease in a particular pregnancy is not always easy. Spectrophotometric estimation of the bilirubin content of a sample of liquor amnii obtained with a needle through the abdominal wall will assist in determining whether haemolysis is occurring and the degree of fetal risk.

Mild cases need no treatment, but in many cases the child requires an *exchange transfusion* after delivery to tide it over until the action of the maternal antibodies ceases. This is done not only to treat anaemia but also to prevent kernicterus. When the vulnerable red cells are replaced the bilirubin level can rise no further, and the exchange also removes some bilirubin. Fresh blood is used at room temperature. For infants with rhesus antibodies the blood must be rhesus negative. In cases with A or B antibodies group O blood, with the plasma replaced with AB plasma and of the same rhesus type as the fetus, is used. After the apparatus has been washed out with a little heparin solution a fine polythene catheter is inserted through the umbilical vein into the vena cava or portal sinus. Then 20 ml of blood is withdrawn and replaced with 20 ml of the donor blood, and the process is repeated until 160 ml/kg has been exchanged. Repeated exchanges may be made if the bilirubin level rises dangerously.

In severe cases, and in those with a history of a previous intrauterine death, delivery at the 35th week or even earlier is sometimes advised to remove the fetus from the action of maternal antibodies. This will give good results only if expert care can be given to the premature baby, including repeated exchange transfusion if necessary.

In a few severe cases, in which it is thought that the fetus will die before it is mature enough to survive delivery, *intrauterine transfusion* may be performed. After ultrasonic localization of the placenta and fetus a needle is passed through the abdominal and uterine walls into the fetal peritoneal cavity, into which packed rhesus negative cells are injected. Absorption is surprisingly complete.

10

Obstetric operations

INDUCTION OF LABOUR

Labour may be started by induction before term, or after term in cases of postmaturity.

Indications

In about 20% of pregnancies one of the following indications for induction will arise, for which reference to other chapters should be made.

1. Pregnancy-induced hypertension.
2. Essential hypertension.
3. Chronic nephritis.
4. Hydramnios.
5. Abruptio placentae
6. Unstable lie.
7. Postmaturity.
8. Diabetes.
9. Haemolytic disease.
10. Anencephaly and other malformations.
11. Fetal death.

With modern methods induction in late pregnancy is nearly always successful, but it must be realized that failure leads to Caesarean section, and with amniotomy there is a small risk of cord prolapse or of infection. If there is any uncertainty about maturity induction may result in the birth of a preterm infant. The indication and risk in each case must be carefully weighed; there is no place for routine induction nor for induction for the convenience of the attendants.

Failure is more likely if the presenting part is not engaged, if the cervix is long, firm and tightly closed, and before the 36th week. If a primigravida needs to be delivered before the 34th week Caesarean section is sometimes preferable to induction.

Methods of induction

The method which is now in general use is to insert a pessary in the vaginal vault which releases prostaglandin E_2 (5 mg) slowly. If uterine contractions do not follow the membranes may be ruptured by passing a small hook ('Amnihook') through the cervix, or with toothed forceps. Scrupulous aseptic technique is essential; anaesthesia is not usually required. A good deal of liquor should be let out, and a final examination made to exclude prolapse of the cord.

If progressive cervical dilatation does not follow at the normal rate (about 1 cm per hour) an intravenous Syntocinon infusion is started. Two units are added to 500 ml of dextrose solution and this is run at 40 drops per minute. The rate of the drip is regulated according to the uterine contractions, which must be carefully observed. Fetal death or uterine rupture can occur if the drip is not carefully supervised, and the method is only suitable for hospital practice. Automatic machines are available which regulate the infusion according to the rate of the contractions, but any ordinary drip can be used so long as the control is accurate. A tocograph and fetal scalp electrode are especially useful for monitoring these cases.

VERSION

External version

This is employed to correct a transverse lie (p. 127) or a breech presentation (p. 121).

Internal version

In the past many obstetric difficulties were overcome by passing a hand into the uterus, turning the fetus and applying traction to the feet (podalic version). Today internal version is rarely employed except for a few cases of shoulder presentation or for delivery of a second twin.

DELIVERY WITH THE FORCEPS

History

The Chamberlen family were Huguenots who fled to England in 1569. The forceps were devised by one of them (probably Peter who died in 1631) and the invention was kept secret for about a century.

Description

There are innumerable types of forceps, but only three are in common use:

1. *Long curved forceps* (e.g. Neville's). There are two blades, each with its handle. The blades are inserted separately and then the handles are locked together. Each blade has a cephalic curve (to fit the head) and a pelvic curve.

This type of forceps is used for delivery of the head from the pelvic cavity (mid-forceps delivery). Delivery of the head from above the pelvic brim (high forceps delivery) is dangerous and is not now performed.

The long curved forceps must always be applied correctly to the sides of the head. Because of the pelvic curve the forceps can only be applied in the anterior position — if the head is not in the antero-posterior diameter of the pelvis it must be rotated manually before applying the forceps. This instrument is not used for rotation.

2. *Short curved forceps* (e.g. Wrigley's). These light forceps

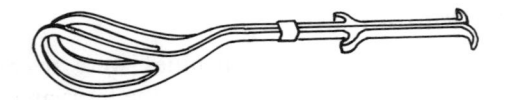

Fig. 10.1 Kielland's forceps.

may be used when the head is on the perineum (low forceps delivery).

3. *Kielland's forceps.* These are of a different design (Fig. 10.1). The pelvic curve is slight and the whole instrument is straighter. The lock allows the blades to slide on each other longitudinally, and (unlike other types) either blade can be inserted first. After correct application to the head the forceps can be used for rotation as well as traction, so that preliminary manual correction is not needed. They are not recommended for use by the inexperienced.

Conditions before application of forceps:

1. The cervix must be fully dilated (except for an occasional case with a small persisting anterior lip of cervix, which can be pushed up after the forceps are on the head). Dangerous haemorrhage from a torn cervix may otherwise occur, or the application may fail.
2. There must be no insuperable obstruction such as that caused by severe pelvic contraction or a tumour. The widest diameter of the head must have passed the pelvic brim.
3. Some malpositions, such as a deep transverse arrest or a mento-posterior position, must first be corrected. The forceps may be used for the aftercoming head during breech delivery.

Indications

1. Delay in the second stage of labour from:
   a. Inadequate uterine action or poor voluntary effort.
   b. Resistant perineum.
   c. Malposition of the head (after correction), e.g. posterior position of the occiput or deep tranverse arrest.
   d. Minor outlet contraction (p. 133).
2. Maternal distress in the second stage
   No patient should be left for more than an hour in the second stage without evident progress. Forceps may be used to assist patients who are exhausted from a long first stage (although this should not have been allowed to occur), and those with cardiac lesions.
3. Fetal distress in the second stage
   This may have no evident cause, or result from prolapse of the cord, hypertension, antepartum haemorrhage or postmaturity.

Maternal dangers

General anaesthesia is dangerous with an unprepared patient and inadequate facilities. The risk can often be avoided by using a pudendal block. Dangerous cervical damage or a third degree perineal tear are unlikely with ordinary care. Failure to deliver with the forceps is usually because of neglect to observe the conditions set out above, and there may then be the hazard of subsequent Caesarean section.

Fetal dangers

Death or cerebral injury may occur from intracranial haemorrhage, and skull fractures can occur. A common injury is facial palsy due to pressure on the VIIth nerve; complete recovery usually occurs.

178 OBSTETRIC ABNORMALITIES

Technique

The lithotomy position is usual, but if a general anaesthetic is used an experienced anaesthetist must be available and the table must be one that can be tilted quickly if the patient vomits. After applying antiseptic cream to the vulva, sterile towels are placed, and the bladder is emptied with a catheter. A vaginal examination is made to determine the position of the head accurately. If the sutures are obscured an ear must be felt. Episiotomy is usually needed.

Before applying ordinary forceps the head is rotated manually, if necessary, so as to bring the occiput to the anterior position. Because of the design of the lock of the forceps the left blade must always be inserted first. This blade is held vertically in the left hand and the fingers of the other hand are used to direct it between the head and the perineum. The handle is then swung down so that the blade passes up to the left side of the pelvis under the guidance of the internal fingers.

The right blade is now passed in a similar way and the handles are locked. If they will not lock easily the blades are not properly applied to the head. They must be removed and reapplied after the head has been correctly rotated.

Traction must be intermittent, and with the pains if they are frequent enough. At first the pull is obliquely towards the floor. As the head descends the handles tend to rise, and the direction of traction is gradually altered so that when the head reaches the vulval orifice the pull is towards the ceiling (Fig. 10.2).

With Kielland's forceps. If the head does not need rotation the blades are applied as already described, but if the head is lying transversely or obliquely the *anterior* blade is selected and inserted first, by passing it into the sacral hollow behind the head and then 'wandering' it around the head until it lies over the anterior ear. The posterior blade is then applied. The head can be rotated with the forceps if necessary.

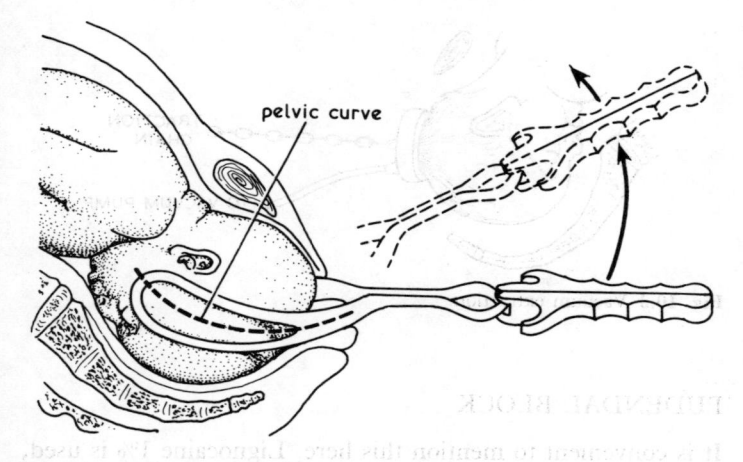

Fig. 10.2 Forceps delivery.

VACUUM EXTRACTOR (VENTOUSE)

This consists of a metal suction cup (supplied in three sizes) which is applied to the fetal occiput. The cup is connected to a vacuum pump by a rubber tube, and there is a chain by means of which traction can be applied to the cup. When a negative pressure (maximum 0.8 kg/cm^2) is produced in the cup the scalp is drawn into it forming a 'chignon', and a firm hold is obtained (Fig. 10.3). Anaesthesia is not required. If the occiput is situated posteriorly it will often rotate during traction. The cup should not be left in place for more than 30 minutes for fear of cephalhaematoma or scalp necrosis.

The ventouse can be used instead of forceps, but in cases of fetal distress forceps delivery may be quicker and therefore preferable. It may also be used in cases of prolonged first stage due to abnormal uterine action when the cervix is more than half dilated, but it should never be used in cases of disproportion.

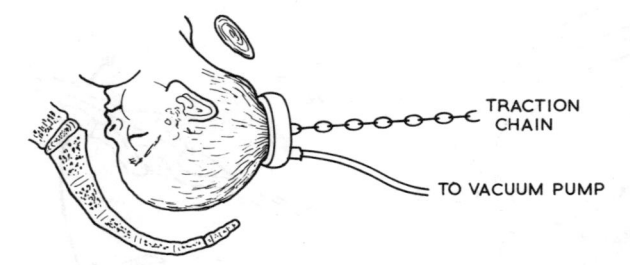

Fig. 10.3 Vacuum extraction.

PUDENDAL BLOCK

It is convenient to mention this here. Lignocaine 1% is used, up to a total of 40 ml. The index finger is placed in the vagina and the ischial spine can then be felt on the side wall of the pelvis. A 10 cm needle is inserted through the vaginal wall to reach a point below and beyond the ischial spine, where 10 ml of solution is injected. The posterior part of the labium majus, which is separately innervated, is also infiltered with another 5 ml of solution. The technique is repeated on the opposite side.

EPIDURAL ANALGESIA

This may also be mentioned here. It is a most effective method of relieving pain, suitable for both normal labour and operative vaginal delivery. It is usually started during the first stage. A needle is inserted into the epidural space by the lumbar route. (The space can also be approached through the sacral hiatus, but such caudal analgesia is now seldom employed). Bupivacaine (Marcain) 0.25% is injected. A polythene catheter is passed through the needle and left in place so that the injection can be 'topped up' as necessary.

Some experience is required in placing the needle and the method is usually in the hands of anaesthetists rather than obstetricians, but whoever is responsible must be able to deal with unexpected complications such as hypotension or temporary respiratory paralysis if the injection inadvertently enters the theca. Uterine tone is normal, or even raised, but voluntary expulsive effort is often impaired, so that low forceps or vacuum extraction is often required.

CAESAREAN SECTION

History

Julius Caesar was not delivered in this way. The name may derive from a Roman law which directed that the child should be removed from any woman who died in childbirth. Various attempts, mostly fatal from haemorrhage or sepsis, were made to perform the operation in the 17th and 18th centuries, but it was not until 1882 that Sänger perfected the classical (upper segment) operation. During labour this was still hazardous from infection until Frank introduced the lower segment operation in 1906.

Indications

These are usually relative and seldom absolute. Factors are often combined, e.g. section might be chosen for breech delivery with an android pelvis, but not for either of these alone. The risk of section is about ten times that of vaginal delivery, but this maternal risk is acceptable for some fetal indications (e.g. breech delivery) if the mother has little hope of a later successful pregnancy because of age, infertility or her obstetric history, whereas in a young normal patient vaginal delivery would be chosen. It is easy to perform a section — the decision when to do it requires experience.

Section is indicated in *some* instances of the following cases. The student will find it instructive to work out the indication in each case.

Maternal and fetal indications

1. Disproportion
2. Pelvic tumours.
3. Malpresentations: breech, brow, shoulder.
4. Abnormal uterine action.
5. Antepartum haemorrhage.
6. Hypertension and eclampsia.

Fetal indications

7. Fetal distress in the first stage of labour, due to prolonged labour, prolapsed cord, placental insufficiency, or sometimes with no explanation.
8. Placental insufficiency; when the fetus is not growing or placental function tests are adverse section is sometimes preferable to induction of labour.
9. Diabetes.

Maternal indications

10. After some operations for prolapse or fistula.
11. Previous Caesarean section. If the section was for a persisting indication (e.g., disproportion) another section is required, but if it was for a non-recurrent indication (e.g., placenta praevia), in spite of a small risk of scar rupture, vaginal delivery in hospital is safer than repeated section.

Preparation

Caesarean section is often an emergency operation during

labour, but elective operations are best performed a week before term.

Purges and enemas are unnecessary. A catheter is passed in the theatre. For premedication, drugs such as morphine, which would depress the fetal respiratory centre, are not used. In emergency cases it has been the practice to give magnesium trisilicate orally to reduce the acidity of gastric contents which might be inhaled, but this is of doubtful benefit, and gastric aspiraton is more effective. All preparations must be completed before the anaesthetic is begun so that the child can be delivered expeditiously.

Blood is taken beforehand for cross-matching, and in cases of placenta praevia blood must be immediately available.

Anaesthesia

Many methods are used by experts. For an elective case a small dose of thiopentone may be followed by nitrous oxide and oxygen, and relaxants (with a cuffed tracheal tube) are often given. Alternatively lumbar extradural anaesthesia is often chosen.

Lower segment operation

This is now the standard procedure. To prevent compression of the inferior vena cava and obstruction to the venous return it is best to have the patient tilted laterally by using a 15° wedge until the baby is delivered. The abdomen is opened through transverse subumbilical incision and a wide Doyen retractor is inserted inferiorly. The peritoneum just above the bladder is incised transversely, and slight downward displacement of the bladder exposes the lower segment, which is also incised transversely. The fetal head is lifted out with the hand or with Wrigley's forceps, and the shoulders are eased out. If the breech presents it is delivered by groin traction.

As soon as the mouth is free it is sucked out; a sterile

attachment to the suction machine should be available. The child is held at the same level as the placenta in the uterus with its head downwards while the cord is divided, and then passed to an assistant. While the placenta is being delivered the anaesthetist gives an intravenous injection of ergometrine 500 micrograms.

The uterine muscle is repaired with two layers of Dexon or chromic catgut, avoiding the endometrium. The uteroversical peritoneum is sutured with fine catgut and the abdomen is closed in the usual way.

Classical section

This is no longer classical, and should simply be called the upper segment operation. It is obsolete except when the lower segment is inaccessible, e.g. from fibroids. The uterus is incised in the midline and the fetus is extracted feet first.

The lower incision is better (even if there is not a well-formed lower segment before labour) because it bleeds less, suturing is easier, and in infected cases there is less risk of general peritonitis. It heals better as it is more quiescent in the puerperium. Subsequent rupture during pregnancy is rare, and rupture during labour is less dangerous than with an upper segment scar.

Sterilization

This may be performed at the time of Caesarean section, but section should never be done just to permit this.

Postoperative care and maternal dangers

The immediate care is the same as that after any laparotomy. The risks are those of any abdominal operation but five are especially important:

1. Anaesthesia in an unprepared patient.
2. Haemorrhage, especially in cases of antepartum haemorrhage.
3. Sepsis, in cases of prolonged or obstructed labour.
4. Pulmonary embolism (p. 162).
5. Rupture of the scar may occur in a subsequent pregnancy or labour. A woman who has had a lower segment section for a non-recurrent indication, e.g. placenta praevia, may have a vaginal delivery (in hospital) in a subsequent pregnancy. A patient whose section was for a persisting indication, e.g. disproportion, would have the section repeated in a subsequent pregnancy, and section is usually repeated if a patient has had two or more sections, and sterilization might then be considered.

Fetal dangers

The fetal mortality after section is relatively high, but in most cases this is because of the indication for the operation (e.g. fetal distress) or prematurity, rather than because of the operation itself.

SYMPHYSIOTOMY

The symphysis pubis can be divided through a small suprapubic incision to allow the pelvic ring to expand slightly. This operation is seldom performed in Britain, but has its advocates in countries where a Caesarean scar may mean disaster in a subsequent unsupervised labour.

DESTRUCTIVE OPERATIONS

These are now seldom required in Britain. *Perforation of the fetal head* is performed only for hydrocephaly (p. 128). In other cases of obstructed labour Caesarean section is safer than craniotomy, even if the fetus is dead. *Cleidotomy* (division of the clavicles) may allow delivery of impacted shoulders with a dead or anencephalic fetus. Other forms of embryotomy are very rarely performed for double monsters, fetal ascites, fetal tumours obstructing delivery, or locked twins (p. 138).

AMNIOCENTESIS

A sample of liquor amnii can be obtained by inserting a needle through the abdominal wall into the uterine cavity. There is a small risk of causing placental bleeding, of introducing fetal red cells into the maternal circulation, or of injuring the fetus. The placental site and fetal position are determined by ultrasound, so that the needle can be directed to avoid them.

Indications

1. In early pregnancy amniotic cells may be grown in tissue culture to detect chromosomal abnormalities, or to determine fetal sex in cases of sex-linked inheritable disease. The incidence of Down's syndrome (trisomy 21) increases with maternal age, reaching 2% in mothers older than 40. In these patients and those who already have a Down's syndrome child amniocentesis may be considered.
2. If the fetus has an open neural tube defect alpha-fetoprotein escapes into the liquor in increased amounts. The discovery of a high concentration in liquor (or in maternal serum) calls for an ultrasonic examination to exclude anencephaly and gross spina bifida.
3. For bilirubin estimation in haemolytic disease (see p. 168).
4. A test for the maturity of the fetal lung is to estimate the lecithin content of the liquor, usually expressed as a ratio

against the sphingomyelin content. The L:S ratio is an index of the surfactant activity of the fetal lung; with a ratio above 2 respiratory distress syndrome is unlikely to occur (p. 192).

CHORIONIC VILLUS SAMPLING

In early pregnancy a fine cannula can be passed through the cervix, or a needle through the abdominal wall, under ultrasound control, to obtain a small sample of chorionic tissue. The trophoblast can be grown in tissue culture for chromosomal analysis, or studied chemically. This allows a quicker diagnosis than is made by culture of amniotic cells.

OXYTOCIC DRUGS

For convenience a note about these is included here.

Ergot

Ergot is a crude extract of a fungus that grows on rye. There are several active substances but the most important for obstetrics is *ergometrine*. The dose of 500 micrograms can be given orally, intramuscularly or intravenously, and the respective times before it acts are about 7 minutes, 4 minutes and ½ minute. The time can be shortened after intramuscular injection by adding hyalase. It causes strong and persisting uterine spasm, and should never be used before the third stage of labour for fear of uteriune rupture or fetal death.

Posterior pituitary extract

Oxytocin (Pitocin) is secreted by the posterior lobe of the pituitary gland, and causes strong uterine contractions in late pregnancy. It has less effect in early pregnancy, and it has little or no effect on the blood pressure, intestine or kidney. Oxytocin is an amino-acid complex which is destroyed in the alimentary tract, and is therefore given by intravenous infusion. This also allows the dose to be accurately controlled. The standard preparation contains 10 units per ml. In small doses it accentuates rhythmical contractions, but large doses can rupture the uterus or kill the fetus. It is used for induction of labour, augmentation of labour or postpartum haemorrhage.

Syntocinon

This is a synthetic preparation which corresponds in action and dosage to oxytocin and is now used in place of it.

Syntometrine

Syntometrine contains 5 units of Syntocinon and 500 micrograms of ergometrine per ml. It is given as an intramuscular injection. The Syntocinon acts after about 3 minutes, and the subsequent action of the ergometrine maintains the uterine contraction.

Prostaglandins

These are a group of long-chain unsaturated fatty acids, originally found in semen but now known to occur in many tissues. Prostaglandin E_2 causes strong uterine contractions when given by intravenous drip, and has been used to induce labour or abortion. Prostaglandins are also absorbed from the vagina. Vaginal pessaries which release PGE_2 slowly are convenient for induction of labour. They are available in forms containing 5 or 10 mg of PGE_2.

11

Care of the newborn child

ASPHYXIA NEONATORUM

Immediately after delivery the establishment of respiration takes precedence over all else. In utero the fetus makes periodic respiratory movements which are sufficient to draw amniotic fluid into the bronchial tree. Immediately after delivery there is mild hypoxia, with a fall in Po_2 and a rise in Pco_2. The respiratory centre of the newborn infant responds to the increased CO_2 concentration, and the response is fortified by a variety of peripheral stimuli, including cold and contact of a catheter on the pharynx. If the infant becomes more severely hypoxic the respiratory centre does not respond to these stimuli (primary apnoea) but after a time irregular gasping respiration occurs, partly due to impulses arising from the carotid and aortic chemoreceptors during oxygen lack. Finally, if the hypoxia is still not relieved the respiratory centre is paralysed and will not respond at all (secondary apnoea).

When respiration is established air is drawn into the alveoli, which expand successively. To expand the lungs not only must their elastic recoil be overcome, but also the tendency of the alveolar walls to cohere. In late pregnancy alveolar cells secrete *surfactant*, a lipo-protein of which lecithin is a main component. This reduces surface tension and allows easier expansion.

As the lungs expand the pulmonary vessels open up, and the ductus arteriosus and the umbilical vessels contract. The ductus and the cord vessels have a natural tendency to contract, and it is believed that high fetal levels of prostaglandins keep them patent until after delivery. As the placental circulation ceases the left arterial pressure rises and the foramen ovale closes.

The infant's respiratory effort is chiefly diaphragmatic, and if the airway is obstructed the sternum will be indrawn with each breath. A negative pressure of 20 cm of water is required for pulmonary expansion.

Aetiology

Failure to breathe soon after birth may be due to:

1. Obstruction to the airway by mucus or meconium.
2. Damage to the respiratory centre by hypoxia before delivery, e.g. from a prolapsed cord, a placental lesion or long labour.
3. Depression of the respiratory centre by drugs such as morphine or pethidine given to the mother within two hours of delivery. Their effect can be counteracted by giving an injection of naloxone hydrochloride 10 micrograms/kg to the infant after birth.
4. Intracranial haemorrhage (p. 200).

Clinical events

Before a breath is taken the infant is cyanosed, but unless the hypoxia is prolonged the pulse rate is more than 100 per minute and the muscular tone is good. If hypoxia is prolonged, either before or after delivery, the circulation fails, the pulse rate is slow, and the blood flow in the skin is reduced so that the infant looks pale. Muscular tone is lost and there is no response to stimuli.

A mark of 0, 1 or 2 may be given for each of these five features: respiratory effort, pulse rate, colour, muscular tone and response to stimuli, and the total gives the 'Apgar score', ranging from 0 to 10.

Treatment

It can be lifesaving to have a doctor experienced in neonatal resuscitation present at the delivery of any infant likely to need this, e.g., preterm infants, cases of fetal distress, Caesarean section, breech or twin delivery.

Immediately after delivery the pharynx and nasal passages are cleared with a soft plastic catheter. Appropriate equipment for further treatment must always be ready. If respiration does not start after clearing the pharynx the baby is placed head downwards on an inclined plane and a laryngoscope is passed. A fine endotracheal tube is inserted and the trachea is cleared by suction. The tube is attached to a water manometer and a suitable supply of oxygen. The lungs are intermittently inflated (for 2 seconds 12 times per minute) at a pressure of 25 cm of water. When spontaneous respiratory efforts begin oxygen is given with a small face mask. If the heart stops external cardiac massage may be tried.

Facilities for chemical control should be available, but acidosis is more often overcome by establishment of respiration than by intravenous (umbilical) administration of alkali and glucose.

In an emergency, with no equipment available, mouth-to-mouth respiration or oral inflation through a fine intratracheal tube are justifiable.

Continuing respiratory distress

Respiratory distress may continue or may first appear some hours after birth. Immediate transfer to a neonatal special care unit is essential. The following conditions require consideration:

Atelectasis

Part or all of the alveoli may be collapsed and airless. This may be a primary condition in small preterm infants. It may occur by secondary absorption of gas beyond bronchioles obstructed by meconium, hyaline membrane or inflammation. Periodic apnoeic phases occur.

Hyaline membrane disease (Respiratory distress syndrome)

In preterm infants and infants of diabetic mothers, a few hours after birth a fibrinous exudate may form in the smaller bronchioles and alveoli. There is a relative deficiency of surfactant in the preterm infant, and this may be increased by hypoxia. With the hypoxia and atelectasis the pulmonary circulation closes down and much of the blood is shunted through the foramen ovale and ductus arteriosus.

Severe respiratory distress occurs, with cyanosis and indrawing of the ribs and sternum. A radiograph shows fine mottling due to patchy atelectasis. The mortality is high, but those who survive to the third day may recover completely.

If there is doubt about the maturity of the fetal lung before delivery the lecithin content of the liquor may be estimated as an indication of the surfactant level. It is claimed that intramuscular injection of dexamethasone (4 mg 6-hourly) to the mother for 2 days before delivery will improve maturation of the fetal lung.

Air accident

Mediastinal emphysema or a pneumothorax may occur. The radiological appearances are obvious, and needling may relieve distress due to pneumothorax.

In the management of all these conditions the administration of oxygen and naso-gastric feeding will be required, sometimes with the correction of respiratory acidosis by intravenous injection of sodium bicarbonate, and the use of antibiotics in cases of infection.

OTHER IMMEDIATE CARE

Eyes and mouth

The eyes and mouth are *not* mopped with wool or gauze; this might introduce infection and certainly would not remove it.

Prevention of hypothermia

In the newborn infant the heat-regulating mechanism is ineffective and it is essential to prevent undue heat loss, either by wrapping the baby in a warm towel and blanket, or in hospital by the use of a radiant heat device. Heat regulation is partly effected by metabolism of brown fat, which is deficient in small infants.

Bathing

The newborn baby is covered with *vernix caseosa*, a cheesy substance consisting of sebaceous secretion with epithelial cells. This should be left alone and the traditional birthday bath should be abandoned. Until the cord has separated cleaning is restricted to the napkin area.

Care of the cord

The cord stump dries and usually separates by granulation in seven days. It is important to prevent umbilical infection and many techniques are in use. One is to tie the cord at about 3 cm with sterile linen thread. A good alternative is to use a sterile disposable plastic clip, which is applied close to the skin and crushes the cord; it can be removed after 48 hours. The stump is left exposed but painted daily with chlorhexidine, 1% in spirit. Chlorhexidine powder may also be applied.

Breast engorgement

The breast may show engorgement in both male and female infants from transfer of maternal oestrogens. No treatment is required.

Examination

Soon after birth the baby is carefully and systematically examined for any congenital abnormality. The passage of urine and meconium is observed. If meconium is not passed in the first 24 hours the rectum is examined. In every case a test for congenital dislocation of the hips is made. On the 7th day a drop of blood is taken for a Guthrie test for phenylketonuria. This is an inherited (recessive) disorder in which phenylalanine is not metabolized and accumulates to cause mental retardation, which is preventable by modification of the infant's diet.

Identification

In hospital every baby should have an identification tape sewn around the wrist.

Prevention of infection

Infants are susceptible to infection. They are best kept separately, each with its mother ('rooming in'), although noisy babies may have to be removed to a nursery. Before any attention the mother or nurse must wash her hands carefully. Any infected baby is isolated.

BREAST FEEDING

A textbook of paediatrics must be consulted for further details. Breast feeding should be encouraged because with it infection is less likely, the composition of the milk is more suitable than that provided by cows, and there are psychological advantages ('bonding') in the close contact of mother and baby. A healthy baby is first put to the breast for a short time immediately after delivery. The baby's cot is kept beside the mother's bed for the first few weeks, and even in hospital on-demand feeding is preferable to a fixed routine. The early feeds may be short and at frequent and irregular intervals, but it is usually found that a regular rhythm of 4-hourly feeds with about 10 minutes at each breast becomes established. For the first 2 days yellow colostrum is secreted (p. 22) which has a high content of protein antibodies.

After feeding on each side the baby is held up to get rid of wind. Before and after feeds the nipples are cleaned with a swab dipped in boiled water.

The best stimulus to lactation is regular suckling. After the 7th day the average requirement is 150 ml of milk per kg of baby per 24 hours. Thirty ml of milk should give 20 calories (4200 J).

Contraindications to breast feeding are few. Rare maternal contraindications are severe cardiac disease, tuberculosis with positive sputum, and puerperal psychosis.

A baby suffering from intracranial injury, respiratory distress or infection may be unable to feed and require tube feeding for a time. Although breast milk is always desirable for them, very small preterm infants may also fail to feed at the breast. Retracted nipples, cleft lip or cleft palate may prevent feeding. For engorgement of the breast see p. 160, cracked nipple, p. 160, and mastitis p. 161. If the baby is to be adopted breast feeding is not attempted.

ARTIFICIAL FEEDING

Cow's milk always contains a wide variety of bacteria and it must always be sterilized for infant feeding. Cow's milk differs in composition from human milk:

	Protein %	Fat %	Lactose %
Human milk	1.25	3.5	7
Cow's milk	3.5	3.5	4.5

The protein is almost all caseinogen and lactalbumin. Cow's milk contains a much larger proportion of the less digestible caseinogen. The fat globules in cow's milk are larger.

Dried milk or evaporated milk preparations are now almost universally used. The drying process partly breaks down the protein, but also destroys vitamins, which must be added. Full-cream preparations have the same fat content as raw milk. Half-cream preparations are made from milk which has been skimmed to remove fat and to which sugar has been added. Low solute preparations which are more sophisticated and more closely resemble breast milk in composition and osmolar qualities are now preferred to half-cream preparations. Paediatric textbooks contain exhaustive (and exhausting) lists of various artificial feeds.

For simplicity:
Feeding is begun with a low solute preparation, made up with water according to the maker's instructions. Starting with 30 ml/kg/24 hours, the amount is gradually increased so that the baby is getting 150/kg/24 hours after about a week. The

feeds may be given 3-hourly at first, but later 4-hourly. A change to a full-cream preparation may subsequently be made.

In hospitals prepacked feeds which only require the attachment of a teat to the bottle may be available.

SMALL INFANTS

It was formerly the practice to designate any baby weighing less than 2500 g at birth as 'premature', whatever the duration of the pregnancy, because records of weight were more likely to be accurate than those of duration. It is now usual to describe these as babies of 'low birth weight'. Two classes are included; babies born before term but of normal weight for the length of gestation, and growth-retarded babies that are 'small-for-dates'. (Some babies fall into both categories.) Tables are available that give the expected range of weights for each week of pregnancy. Growth-retarded fetuses have a higher risk of intrauterine or perinatal death. Babies born before 28 weeks, with an expected weight of less than 1100 g, are regarded as non-viable, although some of them survive. The mortality among babies of low birth weight is high from intracranial haemorrhage, pulmonary complications, infection and feeding difficulties. Kernicterus (p. 169) and haemorrhagic disease (p. 203) may also occur. With babies of between 1100 and 1600 g the mortality is as high as 30%, but with those over 2000 g it is only 3%.

Aetiology and prevention

The incidence of low birth weight is about 7%. No cause is found in a third of the cases, and about half the remainder follow induction of labour. Common causes of the fetus being small-for-dates are hypertension, multiple pregnancy and antepartum haemorrhage. Fetal abnormalities account for

198 OBSTETRIC ABNORMALITIES

a smaller number of cases. The incidence of low birth weight is higher in poorer families and with mothers who smoke heavily.

Improvement is only possible if these causes can be prevented or treated, which is hardly the case at present. If preterm labour is a possibility delivery should be in hospital.

Management

Special medical and nursing experience contributes greatly to success. Paediatric textbooks should be consulted, but immediate treatment includes:

1. *Management of respiratory difficulties.* See p. 191 et seq.
2. *Maintenance of body temperature.* Babies weighing less than 2 kg should be transferred to a special unit. Particular care must be taken not to expose small babies during resuscitation. Small babies are nursed in incubators, where they can be left undisturbed in a moist warm atmosphere (33°C or more) and unclothed to allow free respiration and movement. Larger babies may be in cots, but the room should be kept at 27°C.
3. *Prevention of infection.* Measures include isolation, exclusion of visitors except the parents, careful hand washing, and separate gowns for the attendants at each cot. If there are pulmonary complications prophylactic antibiotics may be given.
4. *Feeding.* Small preterm babies with poor swallowing reflexes can die from aspiration of regurgitated milk. They should not be fed orally until they show sucking movements. A fine polythene tube is passed through a nostril into the stomach. Any gastric fluid is aspirated and feeding can then be begun through the tube. Slightly larger babies who can swallow but not suck effectively are fed with a preterm baby bottle, or from a spoon.

It may take over a fortnight to reach a daily intake of

150 ml of feed per kg weight per 24 hours, and the preterm baby subsequently needs more than this, but there should be no hurry. Two-hourly feeds of diluted expressed breast milk are given at first, and slowly increased to full strength at longer intervals. If breast milk is not available a start may be made with a low solute preparation. Vitamins C and D should soon be added.

5. *Hypoglycaemia.* Small babies, and those with respiratory distress syndrome, may have low glycogen reserves and develop hypoglycaemia. There may be twitching, convulsions, apathy and refusal to feed, and sometimes apnoea. The diagnosis is confirmed by Dextrostix tests on blood from a heel stab. Administration of glucose solution through a naso-gastric tube is usually adequate treatment.

Large babies of diabetic mothers may have hyperplasia of the pancreatic islet and hypoglycaemia because of high blood insulin levels. Early milk feeding may be all that is necessary, but in a few cases small doses of hydrocortisone are required.

6. *Hypocalcaemia.* Small newborn infants may develop twitching and tetany from hypocalcaemia, and the same condition may occur at about the 7th day in infants fed on high-solute artificial feeds. Calcium gluconate may be added to the feeds, or in severe cases given cautiously intravenously.

7. *Kernicterus.* Preterm babies may not be able to conjugate bilirubin effectively, so that severe jaundice occurs with a risk of kernicterus (p. 169). If the serum bilirubin exceeds 340 mmol/l exchange transfusion is required.

BIRTH INJURIES

Cephalhaematoma

A subperiosteal haematoma may occur over a parietal bone. It is limited by the attachment of the periosteum to the edges of the bone. Although absorption is slow and the haematoma may ossify no treatment is required.

Fractures of the skull

These may follow forceps delivery through a contracted pelvis. They may be associated with intracranial haemorrhage. Fractures which remain depressed, or those associated with symptoms, should be elevated surgically and any haematoma evacuated.

Intracranial haemorrhage

1. *Traumatic haemorrhage.* Blood vessels may be torn because of excessive moulding of the head, particularly in cases of disproportion, or of forceps or breech delivery, but the accident can occur with normal labour, especially if it is rapid. If the cerebral vault is displaced upwards by moulding the falx cerebri is under tension. This, or more commonly the tentorium cerebelli to which it is attached, gives way, tearing adjacent vessels.

    Bleeding may occur in various sites:

    Extradural haemorrhage is uncommon except when a large sinus is torn, and then there is usually also subarachnoid haemorrhage.

    Subdural haemorrhage is also uncommon. A small vein is torn between the dura and the arachnoid, and a localized haematoma slowly forms.

    Subarachnoid haemorrhage is the common form of fatal intracranial haemorrhage. If the lateral sinus or the great cerebral vein of Galen is torn the bleeding is subtentorial. Occasionally a tear of the superior longitudinal sinus causes supratentorial bleeding.

2. *Anoxic haemorrhage.* Haemorrhage may also occur in cases of anoxia, especially in preterm infants. A congested

choroid plexus bleeds into the lateral ventricle, or petechial haemorrhages occur widely in the brain substance.

Clinical events

Major haemorrhages may be fatal, minor haemorrhage is undiagnosed. Those of intermediate degree cause difficulty in establishment of respiration, often with pallor and a slow heart rate, and cyanotic attacks. There may be convulsions, twitching, strabismus and failure to suck. The infant may be restless with a persistent high-pitched cry, or drowsy. The fontanelle may be tense, and there may be rigidity of the neck. Recovery may be rapid and complete, or there may be persisting signs of cerebral damage, probably chiefly due to anoxia. An ultrasound scan will show the extent of any intracranial haemorrhage.

In cases of subdural haematoma signs appear slowly over some weeks, with failure to thrive, fits and other local neurological signs. Needling the brain through the fontanelle may prove the diagnosis.

Treatment. Except in cases of subdural haematoma or fracture of the skull bones surgical treatment is not recommended. The infant is disturbed as little as possible. If there are cyanotic attacks oxygen is given. Feeding is postponed for a time, and may have to be by tube. Nursing in an incubator is often convenient. Lumbar puncture is no help, but intracranial pressure can be reduced by the rectal instillation of 50 ml of 10% saline. If the baby is restless intramuscular injections of paraldehyde 0.15 ml/kg may be given.

Nerve injuries

Facial palsy may result from pressure on the VIIth nerve during forceps delivery. Recovery is to be expected.

Brachial plexus injuries are uncommon but may result from

forcible lateral flexion of the head during delivery. In Erb's palsy the 5th and 6th cervical nerves are damaged. Some of the shoulder muscles and the flexors of the elbow are paralysed. The nerves are often stretched rather than completely torn and recovery can be hoped for.

Fractures of the humerus, clavicle or femur

These are rare. With a fractured humerus the arm is strapped to the side, and a fractured femur is strapped to the trunk with the hip fully flexed. Union is rapid and if alignment is bad it soon improves.

Visceral injuries

If hepatic injury is recognized with ultrasound, surgical treatment may be attempted. Adrenal haemorrhage may occur, with severe shock.

SOME OTHER ABNORMALITIES NEEDING EARLY RECOGNITION

The management of most of the following abnormalities will be the responsibility of the paediatrician and *a complete description is not attempted here*, but early suspicion of their presence is important.

Vomiting

Overfeeding or *failure to bring up wind* are simple explanations of most cases, but *obstructive vomiting* needs recognition.

If there is difficulty in swallowing, choking or unusual regurgitation, especially after hydramnios, an oesophageal catheter is passed. If this does not easily enter the stomach immediate investigation for oesophageal atresia or tracheo-oesophageal fistula is required.

Intestinal obstruction may be due to duodenal or ileal atresia, malrotation of the gut or meconium ileus. The last is due to lack of pancreatic enzymes so that undigested meconium forms a putty-like mass. With obstruction there is persistent vomiting, usually bile stained, abdominal distention, visible peristalsis and failure to pass meconium. An X-ray will show dilatation of part of the gut with fluid levels. Surgical exploration is urgently required.

An imperforate anus should be discovered at the first examination.

With a diaphragmatic hernia a lot of the abdominal contents may pass into the chest, and there is both vomiting and cyanosis. Respiratory sounds are absent from one side, and may be replaced by bowel sounds. An X-ray is conclusive.

Symptoms of pyloric stenosis or pylorospasm seldom appear before the second week.

Vomiting may occur with gastroenteritis or other infections.

Diarrhoea

In the young infant this may be due to:

1. Feeding difficulties — feeds which are increased too fast or which contain too much fat or sugar.
2. Infectious enteritis.
3. Parenteral infections such as pyelonephritis.

Haemorrhage

Prothrombin deficiency (haemorrhagic disease). From the 2nd to the 7th day the infant's blood prothrombin level is low, especially in premature infants. Haemorrhage may occur from the stomach (haematemesis) or bowel (melaena), or less commonly in the lungs, brain, skin or elsewhere. An intramuscular injection of phytomenadione (vitamin K_1) 1 mg will allow the liver to form prothrombin until the vitamin is absorbed in the usual way from the bowel.

(Vomiting of blood may occur because the infant has swallowed it from a cracked nipple.)

Umbilical haemorrhage can occur if the ligature is not properly applied.

Thrombocytopenic purpura may be a transient event in the newborn if the mother has this disease.

Uterine bleeding can occur from withdrawal of the effect of the maternal oestrogens.

Jaundice

Physiological jaundice. At birth the infant at term has a high red cell count (more than six million RBC per mm^3) and haemoglobin concentration (16 g per 100 ml). After birth some of the excess red cells are haemolysed. The liver, especially of the preterm infant, may not be able to conjugate all the bilirubin which is released, so that jaundice occurs, starting on about the second day and persisting for a week. The colour is seldom deep, the liver is not enlarged, and the stools are normal.

Natural recovery is to be expected, but cases that do not quickly improve may be helped by whole body exposure to ultraviolet light, taking care to cover the eyes. In preterm infants the bilirubin level may rise dangerously (340 mmol/l) so that there is a risk of kernicterus and exchange transfusion is sometimes required (p. 169).

Infective jaundice. Umbilical sepsis may spread to the liver, or virus hepatitis may occur. Syphilis and toxoplasmosis can affect the liver.

Congenital atresia of the bile ducts causes deep jaundice with pale stools and hepatic enlargement. Surgery may be attempted.

Haemolytic disease. See p. 168.

Other rare causes of jaundice in the newborn include congenital spherocytic anaemia, cretinism, glucose-6-phosphate dehydrogenase deficiency and galactosaemia.

Anaemia

Anaemia is rare as a result of haemolytic disease or haemorrhage (from a slipped cord ligature, division of placental vessels at Caesarean section, or after circumcision).

Infection

The newborn infant has a poor resistance to bacterial infection. This is particularly true of small preterm infants, and with modern intensive care more such infants survive to be at risk. Fulminant multisystemic invasion may occur from infection during labour, or later less acute infection may come from human contacts. Septicaemia or meningitis may occur. Bacterial infection may be with *E. coli*, *Staph. aureus* or streptococci, especially of group B. Viral infections also occur. Symptoms are often misleading or absent, and fever may be slight. Any infection may cause refusal to feed, or vomiting and diarrhoea, and as a result rapid dehydration may occur. Maintenance of fluid and electrolyte balance may require great skill. There should be no hesitation in securing a blood culture or performing a lumbar puncture, and the urine must be carefully examined in every case. It is not possible to wait for the results of bacterial investigation if the baby is very ill. Treatment is begun with a wide-spectrum antibiotic (e.g. cloxacillin 50 mg per kg three times daily) and revised later. All infected infants must be isolated.

Conjunctivitis (ophthalmia neonatorum). Before the introduction of antibiotics there was a serious risk of blindness with gonococcal infection. Today infection is far more often due to staphylococci, chlamydia or other organisms. While bacterial swabs are being examined penicillin eye drops are instilled every 15 minutes for the first 6 hours, and then 3-hourly. Local treatment is given according to the bacteriology. Eye drops are available containing sulphacetamide, penicillin or chloramphenicol, and ointment containing chlortetracycline.

Skin infection. Staphylococci often cause small pustules. Pemphigus is now rare. This used to occur in epidemics and was due to particular strains of staphylococci which caused a generalized eruption of large vesicles containing thin pus. Oral antibiotics are given and the skin is painted with an aqueous solution of gentian violet 1%.

Umbilical infection. Prevention is very important, as infection may spread along the umbilical vein to the liver.

Thrush. Oral infection with *Candida albicans* may occur if the mother has vaginitis. White plaques occur from which the organism is easily cultured. The mouth is painted with nystatin 100 000 units per ml, or with gentian violet 1%.

Pneumonia may follow long labour when organisms are aspirated before or during delivery, or may be due to descending infection from the upper respiratory tract, or to haematogenous spread. Coughing does not occur. Rapid respiration and cyanosis may be seen, but signs are often few unless an X-ray is taken. Infection with group B streptococci from the maternal genital tract may be especially dangerous.

Gastroenteritis. This is extremely dangerous and immediate expert treatment is essential.

Pyelonephritis may cause an obscure illness at the end of the first week, often with vomiting and diarrhoea but not urinary symptoms. An examination of the urine for pus cells should never be omitted.

CARE OF THE NEWBORN CHILD 207

Osteomyelitis may give no local signs at first except that the infant keeps the limb still.

Syphilis. See p. 238.

Convulsions

May be caused by:

1. Cerebral trauma.
2. Infections (e.g. meningitis).
3. Hypoglycaemia, especially in babies of low birth weight or diabetic mothers.
4. Hypocalcaemia (>1.8 mmol/l plasma) especially in artificially fed infants.

12

Obstetric statistics

Reliable obstetric statistics are only available in countries with advanced medical and social services. The following figures only relate to England and Wales.

MATERNAL MORTALITY

The maternal mortality rate is defined as the number of deaths ascribed to pregnancy and child-bearing per thousand total (live and still) births. Deaths from abortion should be included, although they are often tabulated separately. The present rate is about 0.09 per thousand, of which abortion accounts for about 0.006 per thousand.

According to the Confidential Reports of the Ministry of Health in England and Wales (1979–81) the chief causes of maternal death are as shown in the table opposite.

Most of these headings are clear, but one which does not appear in the table is Caesarean section, and no less than 24% of the deaths followed this operation. The risk is calculated to be 0.5 per thousand sections, perhaps because of the indication for the operation, but sometimes because of complications such as pulmonary embolism, haemorrhage or anaesthetic difficulties.

The risk of anaesthesia in obstetrics needs special mention. The operation is often an emergency, and during labour there

Obstetric causes	*Rate per million pregnancies*
Hypertensive disease, including essential hypertension	14.7
Pulmonary embolism	9.4
Anaesthesia, including operations for abortion and ectopic pregnancy	9.0
Ectopic pregnancy	8.2
Haemorrhage (antepartum 2.0, post-partum 3.7)	5.7
Abortion, excluding deaths from anaesthesia	5.7
Sepsis, excluding abortion	3.3
Ruptured uterus	1.6
Other miscellaneous obstetric causes	7.0
Total obstetric causes	72.0
Associated causes	
Illness made worse by or related to pregnancy	37.7
Fortuitous accidents or diseases unrelated to pregnancy	12.7

is gastric retention, with danger of inhalation of gastric contents during induction of anaesthesia. Women in labour must not be given food or fluid by mouth. Anaesthesia should only be induced on a table that can immediately be tipped head-down. An experienced anaesthetist is not always available and a junior may have difficulty in tracheal intubation. Finally, obstetric patients, especially if they have been given relaxants, require full facilities for postoperative observation and care.

In many maternal deaths there was a factor which was largely avoidable, whether due to the doctor, the midwife, the patient, or inadequate facilities. In 18% of cases the patient did not book for care. The commonest medical faults related to the treatment of hypertension or haemorrhage, to anaesthesia, and to the diagnosis of ectopic pregnancy.

FETAL AND NEONATAL MORTALITY

Definitions

A child born before the 28th week is regarded as non-viable and is not included in these statistics (although a number of such infants survive).

Stillbirth. Defined as a child that does not breathe or show any other sign of life. If the heart is beating the child is not stillborn.

Stillbirth rate. Number of stillbirths per 1000 *total* (live and still) births. Present rate about 6.

Neonatal death rate. Number of infants dying during the first year per 1000 *live* births. Present rate about 5.

Infant mortality rate. Number of infants dying during the first year per 1000 *live* births. Present rate about 11.

Perinatal mortality rate. Number of stillbirths and deaths in the first *week* per 1000 *total* births. Present rate under 12. If deaths due to congenital malformations are excluded the 'corrected rate' is about 10.

Causes

As many of the causes of stillbirth may also cause early neonatal death the perinatal mortality is the best index of obstetric care. The cause of a perinatal death can be properly assessed only if both the obstetric history and the autopsy findings are considered. Some causes (e.g. cerebral haemorrhage) may only be proven at autopsy, but on the other hand it is not helpful to list deaths as due to anoxia (from autopsy findings) unless the cause of anoxia (e.g. antepartum haemorrhage) is given. More than one cause may operate, and if the fetus is macerated histological examination may be impossible. There is not space to list all the causes of perinatal death, but the following factors are especially important:

Low birth weight is not a specific cause of death, but often contributes to it.

Congenital malformations account for about 20% of perinatal deaths.

Anoxia. The final cause of fetal death before labour is usually anoxia. This may result from an acute placental lesion such as abruptio placentae, but more gradual placental insufficiency occurs in cases of hypertension and proteinuria. Death before labour may occur with haemolytic disease or diabetes.

Anoxia may also occur during difficult or prolonged labour from interference with placental blood flow by uterine contractions, or from cord compression, or from continuation of the effects of placental lesions already mentioned in the previous paragraph.

Intracranial haemorrhage is often associated with fetal hypoxia, but can itself cause fetal or neonatal death; and other fetal injuries may occur.

Neonatal death may follow events during pregnancy or labour, but in addition respiratory distress syndrome or other pulmonary complications may occur.

Infection, either during delivery or afterwards, accounts for some neonatal deaths and contributes to many more.

In addition to these factors the parity, social status and prior nutrition of the mother will have considerable effect on perinatal mortality.

Provision of better facilities, both of staff and equipment, for neonatal paediatric care is reducing the present perinatal mortality, and by preventing some forms of handicap is preventing much family unhappiness and social distress, and is saving a great deal of money.

SECTION C

Gynaecological disorders

13

Gynaecological investigaton

After hearing the patient's main complaint it is essential to take a full history before any examination, including:

1. History of all pregnancies.
2. Menstrual history, including age of onset, usual cycle and number of days' loss, and irregular or abnormal bleeding, any pain.
3. Enquiry about vaginal discharge, micturition, bowel habit.
4. Any relevant past medical history.
5. Any problems in relation to intercourse, fertility or contraception.
6. Emotional problems in relation to family, housing or occupation.

The patient should empty her bladder before examination. The breasts are examined, and then abdominal examination precedes pelvic examination. The latter is usually performed with the patient in the dorsal position, but the left lateral position is sometimes chosen for an apprehensive patient, or for a virgin in whom rectal examination may be substituted for vaginal examination.

After inspection of the vulva a speculum examination is made with a sterilized bivalve or Sims' speculum. This should precede digital vaginal examination. The bivalve speculum is for use in the dorsal position, and Sims' speculum in the lateral position. The lubricant must be sterile, transparent, and without antiseptic which could interfere with bacteriological examination. A cervical smear is taken with Ayre's spatula and spread on a labelled slide, which is immediately placed in fixative (p. 273). If there is any discharge a little is placed in a drop of saline for direct microscopical examination for trichomonas (p. 245) or monilia (p. 246).

A digital vaginal examination follows. During this examination bimanual palpation is performed by placing the left hand on the lower abdomen and defining the pelvic organs between this hand and the rectal or vaginal finger of the right hand. The position, direction, mobility and size of the uterus and of any other palpable structures are noted.

The history and findings on examination may dictate further tests:

1. Examination of a midstream specimen of urine.
2. Colposcopy and cervical biopsy (p. 273).
3. Endometrial biopsy. Specimens of endometrium can be obtained with a Vabra or other aspirator without anaesthesia, but curettage under general anaesthesia may be preferred.
4. Laparoscopy, including tests for tubal patency (p. 368).
5. Hysteroscopy (p. 369).
6. Ultrasonic examination.
7. Hormonal assays.

14

Embryology and congenital abnormalities

DEVELOPMENT OF THE FEMALE GENITAL ORGANS

We now return to consider the development of the female genital tract in the fetus.

The external genitalia and urogenital sinus

Figure 14.1 shows the tail end of an early embryo. The allantois and hind-gut open into the cloaca, which is subdivided into urogenital sinus and rectum by the down-growth of the septum (S). The two passages are for a time obscured by the cloacal membrane, but when this disappears two separate openings are seen. In front of the cloaca, the genital tubercle

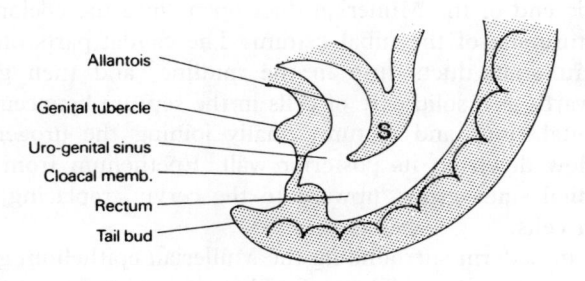

Fig. 14.1 Diagram of sagittal section of hind end of embryo.

217

gives rise to the clitoris, and lateral folds pass back from it on each side to form the labia.

The allantois, which forms the upper part of the bladder, opens into the urogenital sinus; and the urogenital sinus forms the bladder base, urethra and vestibule. The Müllerian ducts grows downwards in the septum (S in Fig. 14.1) between the urogenital sinus and hind-gut, and thus the genital tract comes to lie between the urinary tract and rectum.

The ovary

In the early embryo, the gonad appears on the posterior wall of the coelom as a longitudinal ridge of mesoderm. Primitive sex cells migrate into the gonad from the wall of the yolk-sac.

The genital ridge is continued downwards to the inguinal region, and the gubernaculum appears in it. The ovary descends from its primitive lumbar position, and the gubernaculum persists as the ovarian and uterine round ligaments.

The uterine tube, uterus and vagina

A second ridge appears laterally to the ovary, and in this the Müllerian and Wolffian ducts appear (Fig. 14.2). The cephalic end of the Müllerian duct opens into the coelom at the future site of the tubal ostium. The caudal parts of the two Müllerian ducts fuse in the midline, and then grow downwards as a solid core of cells in the septum between the urogenital sinus and rectum, finally joining the urogenital sinus low down on its posterior wall. Epethelium from the urogenital sinus grows upward to the cervix, replacing this core of cells.

The mesoderm surrounding the Müllerian epithelium gives rise to muscle fibres. The unfused upper ducts become the

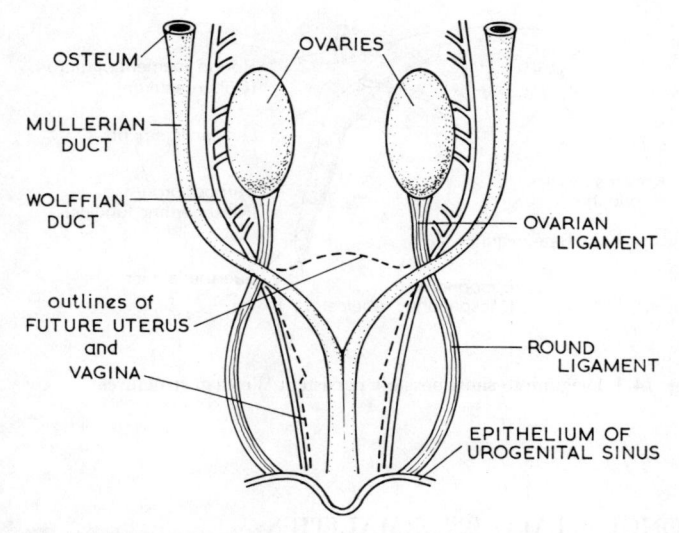

Fig. 14.2 Wolffian and Müllerian tracts.

uterine tubes and the fused ducts below give rise to the uterus and vagina.

Wolffian structures

In the female the Wolffian duct system becomes vestigial, except that at its cephalic end pronephric tubules may persist as small Kobelt's tubules in the outer mesosalpinx, often becoming pedunculated (Fig. 14.3). Epoöphoric and paroöphoric tubules, which may give rise to small cysts, are sometimes found in the mesosalpinx, and represent the mesonephron. A transitory system of tubules (the rete ovarii) lies between these and the ovary.

The Wolffian duct itself may persist, running beside the uterus and vagina, where it is named Gaertner's duct, and may give rise to lateral vaginal cysts.

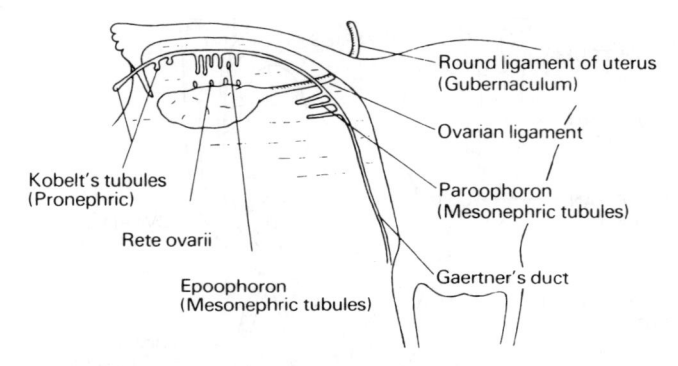

Fig. 14.3 Diagram to show possible persistent Wolffian structures.

CONGENITAL ABNORMALITIES

The ovaries

The ovary may only be represented by a fibrous 'streak' in cases of gonadal agenesis (p. 225) resulting from chromosomal abnormality. There is primary amenorrhoea. No treatment is possible.

Wolffian vestiges

Described above, and of little clinical importance.

The uterine tubes

If the uterus is rudimentary, both tubes may be absent, and with malformation of half of the uterus the corresponding tube may be rudimentary. Accessory abdominal ostia and diverticula occur; the latter may be the site of an ectopic pregnancy.

The uterus

Arrest of development of the whole uterus

The uterus may be rudimentary and only consist of a nodule of fibrous tissue. No treatment is possible.

Imperfect Müllerian fusion

The varying degrees of this condition are best described by illustration (Fig. 14.4).

These abnormalities may cause surprisingly little functional disturbance. If pregnancy occurs in one horn the other empty horn shows hypertrophy and decidual development. In some cases abortion may occur, or obstruction in labour may result from malpresentation or because the non-pregnant horn lies below the presenting part. If recurrent abortion occurs, excision of a medial septum is sometimes successful.

Pregnancy in a rudimentary horn is more dangerous, as the horn ruptures with intraperitoneal bleeding. The symptoms

Uterus didelphys

Uterus bicornis bicollis
Vaginal septum may be absent

Uterus bicornis unicollis

Rudimentary horn

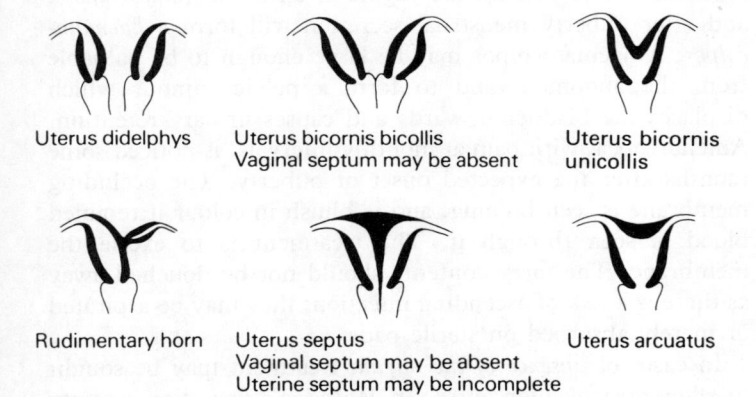

Uterus septus
Vaginal septum may be absent
Uterine septum may be incomplete

Uterus arcuatus

Fig. 14.4 Congenital abnormalities of the uterus.

resemble those of a ruptured tubal pregnancy except that the accident occurs later in pregnancy, often at the 16th week. The treatment is excision of the horn.

In the non-pregnant patient hysteroscopy or hysterosalpingography (p. 369) will assist the diagnosis of these abnormalities.

So-called congenital elongation of the cervix

In this condition, of unknown aetiology, the cervix may extend down to the vaginal orifice, but the fornices are of normal depth. The redundant cervix is amputated.

The vagina

Vaginal septa have already been mentioned. Imperfect Müllerian canalization may occur so that the vagina is absent or shows atresia of varying extent. The commonest site of obstruction is just above the hymen, usually by a thin membrane. If uterine function is normal cervical mucus may accumulate and distend the vagina of an infant (*mucocolpos*), and after puberty menstrual secretion will form a *haematocolpos*. A haematocolpos may be large enough to be palpable from the abdomen, and to form a pelvic tumour which displaces the bladder upwards and causes urinary retention. Amenorrhoea, with pain at monthly intervals, is noticed some months after the expected onset of puberty. The occluding membrane is seen bulging, and is bluish in colour if retained blood is seen through it. The treatment is to excise the membrane. The tarry contents should not be douched away as there is a risk of ascending infection; they may be aspirated or merely absorbed on sterile pads.

In cases of *absence of the vagina* treatment may be sought to allow normal intercourse. In McIndoe's operation a cavity is dissected at the site of the vagina, and a suitable mould carrying a Thiersch skin graft is inserted and stitched in place for several weeks to prevent contraction of the cavity. In Williams's operation, which is simpler, the posterior parts of the labia are sutured together so as to form a tubular recess.

Abnormalities of the urinary tract

In cases of congenital abnormalities of the uterus or vagina intravenous pyelographs often show urinary abnormalities such as double ureter, or absence of the kidney on one side.

SEXUAL DETERMINATION

In cases of abnormal anatomical development the determination of sex may be difficult. It is usual to define the sex by the type of gonad present, but uncertainties arise when the gonads are of mixed type or undifferentiated, and the configuration of the body (phenotype) and the form of the external genital organs may not correspond to the sex of the gonads. Even in individuals of normal physical and endocrine development abnormalities of psychology and behaviour may arise.

Basic sexual differentiation is determined by the genes, which are parts of the nuclear chromosomes. There are normally 46 chromosomes in each cell of the human body. In the reduction division during maturation of the sex cells these chromosomes divide into 23 pairs, so that each ovum or sperm contains half the ordinary complement. Forty-four of the chromosomes (the autosomes) divide into pairs that appear identical, but two of the chromosomes (the sex chromosomes) show specialization. In the female the sex chromosomes consist of paired XX chromosomes, so that after the reduction division every ovum contains an X chromosome. In the male the sex chromosomes consists of an X chromosome and a small Y chromosome, so that after the reduction division half the sperms will contain an X chromosome and half a Y chromosome. Conjugation of sperms and ova give rise to XX and XY pairs again.

Every normal body cell has this male or female constitution. Cells which contain two XX chromosomes have a nodule of chromatin which can be seen with the microscope, and represents one (inactive) X chromosome. (Abnormal cells with more than two X chromosomes may have more than one visible chromatin nodule.) The Y chromosome can be identified by immunofluorescent microscopy. Observations are usually made on polymorphonuclear leukocytes or cells scraped from buccal epithelium. It should be realized that it is the invisible genes which determine sex, and these are not only found in the sex chromosomes but are scattered among the autosomes; yet the visible chromosomal pattern is a useful laboratory test that gives at least a partial indication of the genetic pattern.

In normal females the combined influence of the genes of the paired XX chromosomes and of the autosomes causes development of the cortex of the gonad to form an ovary, and the development of the Müllerian system. In normal males, with XY chromosomes, the genes cause suppression of the development of the cortex of the gonad and the medulla develops into a testis, while the Wolffian system predominates. The development of the gonad seems to be determined by the primitive germ cells that migrate into it from the region of the yolk-sac in early embryonic life. The gonad ultimately establishes a male or femal hormonal pattern, which causes the sexual changes of puberty.

Animal experiments suggest that in a male fetus the hypothalamus is 'imprinted' by male sex hormones. In a female after puberty the hypothalamus will release GnRH cyclically, but in a male fetus this pattern is abolished by male sex hormone and the hypothalamus eventually has a non-cyclic release pattern.

Abnormal sexual differentiation and intersex

The ill-defined term intersex is applied to patients in whom the diagnosis of their sex is difficult. Some have chromosomal abnormalities, in some there is failure of development of the gonad or its response to hormones is defective, or there may be abnormal hormone metabolism. Abnormal psychological orientation is not usually caused by chromosomal or hormonal defects.

Gonadal agenesis

This term is applied to patients with female phenotype (body form) in whom the ovaries are only represented by fibrous streaks. There is no breast development. Those with *Turner's syndrome* are often of short stature, and may have associated congenital abnormalities, including a web-like skin fold on each side of the neck, cubitus valgus and coarctation of the aorta. Most of these individuals have 45 chromosomes, and it is thought that one X chromosome is missing.

Other patients who are tall or of normal stature, with streak ovaries, female phenotype but absent breast development, have been described as cases of *simple gonadal agenesis* or *mixed gonadal agenesis*. The chromosomal pattern of the former may be 46 XX or 46 XY, and of the latter a mosaic of 46 XX and 46 XY. It is thought that in some cases the Y chromosome is defective, but in others the reason for failure of development of the gonad is unknown. It may be noted that absence of breast development with a female phenotype is suggestive of gonadal agenesis. The gonadal hormones are absent and there is primary amenorrhoea.

Klinefelter's syndrome

This only concerns the gynaecologist in the course of investigating male infertility. The body form is male, with small but normal external genitals, but usually azoospermia. These individuals have 47 chromosomes, a nuclear nodule is present, and the structure is XXY.

True hermaphroditism

This is rare, but cases have been described with a testis on one side and an ovary on the other, with predominant development of Mülerian and Wolffian tracts on the corresponding sides, or there may be ovotestes. The patients are infertile, and the chromosomal pattern may be of either type or a mosaic.

Testicular feminization (androgen insensitivity syndrome)

In this condition, which may be familial, the body form is feminine, often tall, with well-formed breasts but no pubic hair. There is amenorrhoea, and testes are found instead of ovaries. The chromosomal pattern is that of a normal male, 46 XY. Testosterone is present in normal amounts, but for some unknown reason the tissues do not respond to it. As there is a risk of disgerminoma (p. 290) arising in the gonads, these are removed after puberty.

Adrenogenital syndrome

This is a familial disorder in which the adrenal cortex fails to convert progesterone into cortisol normally. Cortisol normally inhibits the production of adrenocortical hormone by the pituitary gland, but in this disease the output of ACTH is unchecked, so that the abnormal adrenal cortex is overstimulated, and it responds by excessive production of androgens (it is unable to respond by producing cortisol as a normal gland would). A female child may have a large clitoris and a cloacal membrane so that the external organs resemble those of a male, although the internal organs are normal. The androgens cause masculinizing effects, and at a later stage there is amenorrhoea, hirsutes and excessive muscularity. There is an increased urinary output of 17-oxosteroids, pregnanetriol and pregnanetriolone. The condition is reversible by giving cortisol, which inhibits the excessive output of ACTH.

Management of cases of intersex

In a child full investigation is essential, including chromosomal studies, oxosteroid and other hormonal estimations, pelvic examination under anaesthesia, and occasionally laparoscopy. Diagnostic problems include that of a male child with hypospadias and undescended testes. It is important that a child is brought up in the correct sex, and treatment is occasionally possible, e.g. for adrenogenital syndrome, or by surgical modification of anatomical abnormalities. Oestrogens will effect breast development.

In general the body form will determine the way an individual is brought up, and in older patients there is little purpose in altering the patient's mode of life, whatever the scientific sex may be.

15

Pelvic injuries and displacements

Most gynaecological injuries follow childbirth, and prevention and immediate treatment is the duty of the obstetrician.

Vulval and perineal injuries

Direct injury may cause lacerations or a vulval haematoma (see p. 147). Very rarely a hymeneal tear may bleed enough to need suture. Obstetrical perineal tears are described on p. 148.

Vaginal lacerations

Apart from rare injuries at coitus, these nearly always follow delivery, and accompany a perineal tear.

Vesicovaginal fistulae

These may be caused by obstetrical or surgical injury, or less commonly by ulceration of a cervical or vaginal carcinoma.

Obstetrical injury may be immediate, by unskilful use of instruments, or delayed, when ischaemic sloughing follows pressure during unduly prolonged labour. Operative injuries may occur at hysterectomy or colporrhaphy.

Vesicovaginal fistulae cause incontinence which is usually complete, but may be partial with small fistulae. The deep red bladder mucosa can be seen through a large opening, but small fistulae may only be found by cystoscopy or injecting methylene blue into the bladder. Fistulae are often complicated by extensive scarring and by secondary cystitis and vulvo-vaginitis.

Most traumatic fistulae can be closed by a vaginal operation. The vesical mucosa and vaginal epithelium are freed and sutured separately. Afterwards the bladder is kept drained with an indwelling catheter. In a difficult case a suprapubic cystotomy may be required, or an abdominal approach to the fistula. When all else fails the vagina can be closed surgically below the fistula (colpocleisis).

Rectovaginal fistulae

These usually follow childbirth, but can also be due to neoplasm or radium burns. Recent obstetrical fistulae sometimes heal spontaneously; otherwise they are repaired by freeing the rectal mucosa and vaginal epithelium and suturing them separately.

Cervical injuries

Minor cervical tears occur in every labour, but severe tears expose the cervical mucosa (ectropion), and the exposed mucosa gives rise to discharge. Incompetence of the cervix, as a result of a tear involving the internal os, or damage by injudicious surgical dilatation, may be a cause of miscarriage. Large tears require repair (trachelorrhaphy).

Injuries to the body of the uterus

Apart from obstetrical rupture of the uterus (p. 149), the only common injury is perforation during dilatation and curettage, or during attempts to abort pregnancy. Perforation with a small instrument such as a sound is seldom dangerous unless the uterus is infected, or contains new growth, or unsterile instruments are used. In most cases it is only necessary to keep the patient under observation for a few days, and laparotomy is only needed if there is a large tear, and particularly if bowel is seen.

DISPLACEMENTS OF THE UTERUS AND VAGINA

A few anatomical facts may first be mentioned:

The supports of the uterus

It is strongly emphasized that the broad ligaments are only peritoneal folds, and that the direction of the round ligaments is such that they cannot support the uterus. The real uterine supports are the cardinal and uterosacral ligaments, which are condensations of the visceral pelvic fascia (Fig. 15.1). Each *cardinal ligament* (transverse pelvic ligament) extends from the side wall of the pelvic cavity near the arcus tendineus to the supravaginal cervix and vaginal vault. It is a fan-shaped sheet of fascial tissue, containing numerous blood vessels, and with the ureter running forward between its upper fibres. The

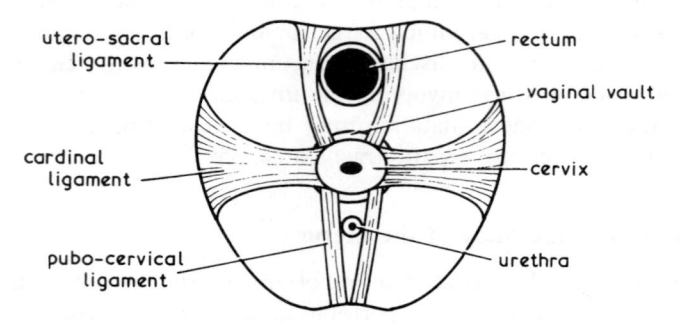

Fig. 15.1 Diagram of pelvis (from above) to show pelvic ligaments.

medial end of the ligament is closely related to the uterosacral ligament. The uterosacral ligaments pass from the sacrum to the cervix. The rectum and the rectovaginal peritoneal pouch lie between them.

The supports of the vagina

The anterior and posterior vaginal walls are in contact, and anything that supports the posterior wall will therefore support the anterior wall. The lowest third of the posterior wall rests on the perineal body, into which levator ani and the superficial perineal muscles are inserted. With its fellow of the opposite side levator ani forms a sling which draws the perineal body forwards and upwards, and so supports the vaginal walls and bladder. The urethra and vagina pass forward between the medial edges of the levator muscles, and some of the muscle fibres are inserted into them (Fig. 3.3).

Prolapse

This term is applied to descent or protrusion of the vaginal walls or uterus.

Aetiology

Prolapse is the result of weakening of the pelvic supports which have just been described. In 99% of cases the patients are parous. During pregnancy the structures are hyperaemic and softened, and during labour the perivaginal fascia may be stretched or torn. If pregnancies are repeated at short intervals, with inadequate rest after each one, the supports will have little chance to recover.

After the menopause the pelvic structures atrophy, and prolapse not infrequently first appears then. Such atrophy is always the cause of the rare cases in nulliparae.

232 GYNAECOLOGICAL DISORDERS

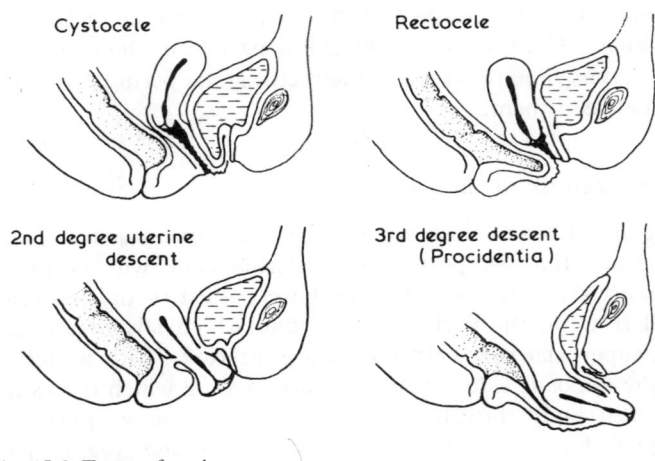

Fig. 15.2 Types of prolapse.

Increased intra-abdominal pressure or persistent coughing may be contributory factors.

Anatomy

The lesions may be artificially subdivided:

1. *Uterine descent.* Descent of the uterus can only occur if the cardinal and uterosacral ligaments are stretched. The perineal body does not directly support the uterus, but if it is deficient the vaginal walls are unsupported, and may prolapse. The vagina may prolapse first, or the uterus may descend first and the vaginal walls follow. Once vaginal drag begins the supravaginal cervix becomes elongated by traction; while the vaginal cervix becomes oedematous, often with secondary infection or ulceration. Degrees of descent are: First, retroversion with descent of the cervix to the vaginal orifice. Second, cervix protruding. Third (or procidentia), uterus outside the vulva with complete vaginal inversion. In

procidentia the prolapsed mass contains bladder, uterus and adnexae, peritoneal pouches which may contain gut, and drawn down rectal wall.

2. *Anterior vaginal wall descent (cystocele).* This occurs with uterine descent, but can occur alone. The bladder fails to empty completely at micturition, and cystitis often occurs.

3. *Posterior vaginal wall descent (rectocele).* If the perineal body is damaged the lower part of the posterior wall can prolapse, together with a pouch of the underlying rectal wall. The upper part of the posterior vaginal wall inevitably descends if the uterus descends.

4. *Hernia of the recto-vaginal pouch (enterocele)* This often accompanies a rectocele, but may occur alone. This is a type of prolapse which may occur after vaginal hysterectomy or repair if the structures at the vaginal vault are inadequately opposed. It is an uncommon sequel of abdominal hysterectomy.

Symptoms

There is a sensation of perineal weakness — sometimes described as 'bearing down'. Urinary symptoms include frequency, stress incontinence (p. 352) and, only in cases of procidentia, retention. Discharge may come from an exposed and oedematous cervix. Backache is occasionally relieved by treatment of prolapse, but is far more often found to be due to other causes.

Treatment

Surgical treatment is recommended (see p. 355).

Treatment with a pessary is only palliative, never curative, and is inconvenient as the patient must have the pessary changed at intervals. It may occasionally be recommended for a patient who is unfit or too old for operation, or as a temporary expedient in early pregnancy or for a young woman who hopes for a further pregnancy.

Ring pessaries are made of plastic material. The ring is compressed for insertion, and should be large enough to fill the vaginal vault, but should never cause discomfort. A ring is useless if the vaginal orifice is too relaxed to retain it, and often fails to control a cystocele. Pessaries will not relieve stress incontinence.

Pregnancy after an operation for prolapse

In most cases vaginal delivery with episiotomy is recommended, but if stress incontinence has been successfully cured Caesarean section may be considered.

Retroversion

In retroversion the uterine fundus is directed backwards and the cervix is directed forwards. On vaginal examination the body of the uterus is felt through the posterior fornix, and cannot be felt bimanually. *Retroversion is a physical sign, not a disease.*

Clinical varieties

'*Congenital retroversion*'. This is not congenital, but arises at puberty; when the uterus enlarges it may fall backward instead of becoming anteverted. About 20% of healthy women have retroversion of this type, which does not give rise to symptoms, nor require treatment.

If pregnancy occurs the retroverted uterus nearly always rises up uneventfully, but rarely becomes incarcerated in the pelvis (see p. 95).

Puerperal retroversion. At postnatal examination the uterus may be found to be retroverted, but if there are no symptoms, or if the retroversion is known to have been present before pregnancy, then no treatment is required. Even if there is backache this is more likely to be due to poor posture and fatigue than to the retroversion. Dyspareunia occurs in very few cases. Treatment is usually pointless.

Retroversion secondary to other pelvic lesions. Fixed retroversion may be caused by adhesions from salpingitis, pelvic peritonitis or endometriosis. The prolapsed uterus is retroverted. In all these cases there may be symptoms, but these are not due to the retroversion, which is only incidental.

Treatment

Retroversion can be corrected by the operation of ventrosuspension in which the round ligaments are used to hold the uterus forwards. This is occasionally performed for dyspareunia, particularly as part of an operation for endometriosis or chronic salpingitis. The ligaments are plicated, either by open operation or by a laparoscopic technique.

Chronic inversion of the uterus

In inversion the uterus is turned inside out, and when it is complete the uterine fundus passes through the cervix to lie in the vagina, while the tubes and ovaries are dragged down into the cup formed by the inverted uterus. Acute inversion is a dangerous obstetrical accident (p. 152). Very rarely such cases persist as chronic inversion. It may also occur from traction on a fundal fibromyoma or sarcoma as the uterus contracts to expel the tumour.

Chronic inversion causes pain and bleeding. The cervix forms a tight constriction ring so that replacement is difficult. Operations to divide the ring are possible, but vaginal hysterectomy is usually preferable.

16

Infective diseases

SEXUALLY TRANSMITTED DISEASES

Recently there has been a great increase in the number of cases of sexually transmitted disease. Conditions encountered in special clinics include, in rough order of frequency, chlamydial and non-specific genital infection, candidiasis, gonorrhoea, genital warts, trichomoniasis, herpes genitalis, pubic lice, syphilis and scabies. Diseases less commonly encountered include molluscum contagiosum, chancroid, lymphogranuloma venereum, granuloma inguinale, hepatitis and acquired immune deficiency syndrome. Some of these conditions are met in ordinary gynaecological clinics: see candidiasis (p. 246), trichomoniasis (p. 247), vulval warts (p. 242), and molluscum contagiosum (p. 242). The following account relates only to the aspects of venereal disease occurring in women. For the effects of these diseases in pregnancy see p. 107.

Gonorrhoea

The gonococcus is a Gram-negative diplococcus found in the pus cells from lesions. Gonococci infect the epithelium of the urethra, vestibular (Bartholin's) glands and cervix, but not the thick vaginal epithelium of the adult. The infection spreads in the submucous tissues, causing acute inflammation with purulent discharge. It may spread upwards to the endometrium and tubes, and rarely by the blood stream to joints or the iris. Gonococci may cause ophthalmia neonatorum and rarely vulvo-vaginitis in children.

Symptoms and signs

The incubation period is from 2 to 5 days. In women symptoms may be slight, but purulent urethral and cervical discharge may occur, with frequency of micturition. Lower abdominal pain or fever suggest spread to the tubes or pelvic peritoneum. Bartholin's glands may be swollen and tender, with the duct orifices evident as red puncta. If there is profuse discharge this is often caused by coincidental trichomoniasis. The local symptoms resolve spontaneously, but cervicitis and salpingitis may persist.

Diagnosis

In the acute stage bacterial smears and cultures are taken from the urethra and cervix after wiping away gross discharge. Cultures are best put up immediately on warm serum agar, but alternatively swabs can be sent to the laboratory in Stuart's transport medium.

Treatment

A variety of antibiotics are usually effective. A single dose of ampicillin 2 g, with oral probenecid 1 g may be chosen. If the organism is resistant an intramuscular injection of spectinomycin is given. Local treatment is not required, but there should be no intercourse until follow-up tests are negative. To confirm cure, swabs are taken just after the next two menstrual periods. A serological test for syphilis is done at the last examination. Male contacts should be traced and investigated.

Chlamydial infection

'Non-specific urethritis' has long been recognized in males. Many of these cases have been shown to be caused by *Chlamydia trachomatis*, but a different strain from that which causes trachoma. In women attending VD clinics this organism can frequently be found in the cervix or urethra. The only symptom may be slight cervical discharge, but some cases of salpingitis are caused by *Chlamydia*. Bacterial diagnosis is difficult. The organism is an obligatory intracellular parasite, and will only grow in cell culture. Immunofluorescent serum antibody tests are available.

Treatment with tetracycline or erythromycin is effective, and should be given if the consort has urethritis.

Chlamydia can also cause ophthalmia neonatorum (p. 206) and lymphogranuloma venereum (p. 240).

Herpes genitalis

Vulval infection with herpes II virus causes a vesicular eruption with burning, itching and dysuria. Cervical infection may also occur. Recurrent attacks are very common. Acyclovir 200 mg orally 5 times daily for 7 days will reduce the severity of the attack, but does not seem to prevent recurrent attacks.

Herpes which is active during delivery may cause dangerous fetal infection, and in such a case Caesarean section is preferable to vaginal delivery.

Herpes virus has been found in association with some cases of cervical carcinoma, but is not generally believed to cause it.

Syphilis

This serious disease is caused by *Treponema pallidum* and is sexually transmitted, except that a fetus may be infected from its mother.

The *primary chancre* is often unnoticed in women. It may occur anywhere in the lower genital tract, and occasionally on the anus, lip, nipple or finger. After an incubation period of 10–90 days (usually 28) an indurated papule appears, which breaks down to form an almost painless ulcer with firm margins, which persists for 3–4 weeks. The inguinal glands show painless, discrete, firm enlargement. Secondary infection may confuse any of these signs. The serological tests do not become positive until 6–12 weeks after infection.

In the *secondary stage*, after about 2 months, malaise, anaemia, limb pains and slight fever may occur, with widespread enlargement of lymphatic glands. Eruptions appear on the skin and mucous membranes, with patchy pigmentation and alopecia. Many types of non-irritating rashes occur, including papules, pustules and scaly eruptions. White 'mucous patches' are seen on the buccal mucosa, in which thick grey epithelium separates to leave shallow ulcers. Condylomata lata occur on the vulva and perineum as broad flat patches of white sodden epithelium.

In the *tertiary stage* serious lesions of bones and joints, heart and blood vessels, nervous system and eyes may occur.

Diagnosis

In the primary stage suspicious ulcers are examined for treponemata. After cleaning the surface with saline, any serum that exudes is examined by the dark-ground method. Treponemata may also be found in lymph aspirated from a gland. After 6–12 weeks the serological reactions such as the VDRL (venereal disease reference laboratory) test, and treponemal haemagglutinin assay tests, become positive.

Treatment

A typical course of treatment consists of 10 consecutive daily injections of 600 000 units of delayed-action penicillin. If the patient is sensitive to penicillin, tetracycline 500 mg 6-hourly for 21 days may be used, or erythromycin in similar doses. Supervision is maintained for at least 2 years, or until the serological tests are negative. Sexual transmission becomes improbable after 2 years, even without treatment, but a woman can infect her child *in utero* for a longer period.

Soft sore (Chancroid)

This is caused by *Haemophilus Ducreyii*, a small Gram-negative bacillus that is difficult to culture. One to 4 days after intercourse multiple painful vulval ulcers appear. The inguinal glands are swollen, matted and often suppurate. The disease responds to several antibiotics, including chlortetracycline and cotrimoxazole.

Lymphogranuloma venereum

This disease, rare in Britain, is caused by certain strains of *Chlamydia*. The initial lesion is vesicular, but granulomatous masses appear later, with eventual fibrosis and ulceration. The inguinal glands may suppurate. Rectal infection and stricture may occur, and epithelioma is an occasional sequel. Chlortetracycline or chloramphenicol are effective for treatment, and aspiration of abscesses or excision of infected tissue may be necessary.

Granuloma inguinale

A venereal disease seen in tropical countries. In the cells of the granulomatous lesions capsulated bacteria (Donovan bodies) are found. Ulceration and scarring may involve the whole vulval area. The disease responds to streptomycin or tetracycline.

Acquired immune deficiency syndrome

AIDS was first recognized in 1981. It is still relatively uncommon in women in Britain, but public concern justifies a fairly full description. It is caused by retrovirus HTLV III (human T-cell lymphotrophic virus). The virus is present in the blood of infected patients, from which transmission can occur into the blood of other individuals. It may also be present in semen. Within 2 or 3 months of infection antibodies to the virus are formed. Many patients with antibodies remain well, but in some cases immune deficiency arises because the virus invades T4 lymphocytes, so that a variety of bacterial infections such as pneumonia and septicaemia occur. It ultimately infects brain cells, causing encephalopathy.

The infection is commonly transmitted to males during homosexual rectal intercourse, probably through anal abrasions. It is much less frequently transmitted to women during normal vaginal intercourse. It can be transmitted by infected needles during intravenous drug abuse. Transmission has occurred by blood transfusion and to haemophiliacs during treatment with blood products, but donor blood is now discarded if antibodies are present and blood products are heat-treated. The virus can be transmitted to the fetus in utero, and to an infant in breast milk.

It is not conveyed by casual or non-sexual contact, but finding a positive antibody test raises difficult ethical questions. If the patient is informed, severe anxiety may be caused, but if he or she is not informed, sexual partners may be at risk. Contracts of employment or insurance may be threatened. There is at present no treatment.

VULVITIS

Specific infections

1. Infection with *Candida albicans* (monilia) is common. It

may occur when there is glycosuria in diabetes or pregnancy, but also in other patients. It is sometimes, but not always, sexually transmitted. The vulva is acutely inflamed, and white patches occur in which the mycelium is found. It may be treated with nystatin vaginal pessaries (100 000 units) and cream. There are many other effective local applications, e.g. clotrimazole (Canesten).
2. *Herpes genitalis.* See p. 238.
3. *Vulval warts* (condylomata acuminata) are caused by human papillomavirus (HPV), which may be sexually transmitted. The warts are usually multiple and may also occur in the vagina and on the cervix. They are treated by coagulation with diathermy, by cryosurgery, or with a laser.
4. *Molluscum contagiosum* is caused by a virus which is transmitted by contact. White umbilicated nodules may occur anywhere on the body. On the vulva they can be treated with diathermy, cryosurgery or a laser.
5. *Primary chancre.* See p. 239.
6. *Chancroid.* See p. 240.
7. *Lymphogranuloma venereum.* See p. 240.
8. *Granuloma inguinale.* See p. 240.

Secondary vulvitis

Occurs in cases of:

1. Vulval irritation from scratching (see pruritus).
2. Profuse vaginal discharge from any cause.
3. Urinary incontinence, especially with pyuria.
4. Diabetes, when candida grows in the excreted sugar.

Leukoplakia, primary atrophy and chronic vulvitis

Dermatologists are very critical of the use that gynaecologists have made of the terms leukoplakia and kraurosis in the past, but modern attempts to include all these conditions under the single heading of 'vulva dysplasia' are unhelpful. The following description tries to use dermatological terms correctly. For diagnosis biopsy and the help of the skin specialist may be necessary.

1. Any persistent vaginal discharge will cause pruritus, and scratching may cause *lichenification* of skin. Adjacent parts of the perineum and thighs may be involved. Inflammatory changes cause thickening and and oedema of the skin (not to be confused with true leukoplakia). The treatment is to cure the discharge, to give sedatives which are adequate to secure sleep, and local antipruritics to stop the scratching, such as zinc cream with 1% phenol. Anaesthetic creams (e.g. benzocaine) may be used, but there is some risk of sensitivity reactions. Hydrocortisone ointment (1%) is often helpful.
2. *True leukoplakia* (hypertrophic dystrophy) occurs in patches, but is confined to the vulva. There is severe pruritus. The involved skin is white and thickened. Epithelial proliferation occurs, with irregular downgrowth of papillae, and heaping up of swollen surface cells. Hyaline degeneration occurs in the collagen fibres in the dermis. *In many cases epithelioma follows*, and leukoplakic skin should be excised without delay.
3. *Lichen sclerosus* is commonly mistaken for leukoplakia. Lesions may extend back to the anus. Soreness and pruritus occur. There are ivory coloured papules, with hyperkeratosis around hair follicles. The cause is unknown and treatment is symptomatic.
4. *Primary atrophy* (kraurosis) is usually seen in postmenopausal women, whose complaint is of pain. The skin is atrophic, thin and dry, with a yellow or red colour. Shrinking of labia and contraction of the vaginal orifice ultimately occur. Some of these cases respond to oestro-

gens (ethinyl oestradiol 10 micrograms orally daily and local applications of dienoestrol cream).

Pruritus vulvae

Vulval irritation is caused by:

1. Urinary conditions: glycosuria, pyuria, incontinence.
2. Vaginal discharge from any cause.
3. Rectal conditions: haemorrhoids, threadworms.
4. Skin diseases: leukoplakia, lichen sclerosus, nits, scabies, allergic reactions, etc.
5. In many cases there is a psychosomatic factor.

Vulval irritation is maintained by scratching, and not infrequently by applications prescribed for treatment.

Treatment

The cause must be sought and removed. In the meantime sedatives and local antipruritics are given to stop the scratching, such as coal tar lotion, phenol 1% in zinc cream, or gentian violet 1% solution for cases with sepsis. Hydrocortisone ointment 1% is used in cases due to sensitization. Oil, rather than soap and water, should be used for cleansing. In resistant cases local injection of proctocaine in oil has been used, and a laser may be employed to destroy the superficial epithelium and nerve endings.

Bartholinitis (infection of vestibular gland)

The vestibular glands of Bartholin lie on either side of the vaginal orifice, and are compound racemose glands with cubical epithelium. The orifice of the duct is medial to the labium minus and superficial to the hymen.

Acute Bartholinitis may occur in gonorrhoea, but is far

more often the result of infection by other organisms. There is local pain, and pus can be seen coming from the duct. A Bartholin abscess may follow, as a tender hot swelling under the posterior part of the labium minus. Systemic antibiotics, and drainage by excision of a small ellipse of skin which includes the site of the duct, are required. Such abscesses tend to recur, and then the gland is excised, leaving the wound widely open to drain.

VAGINITIS

The vagina has a wall of smooth muscle and a rugose lining of squamous epithelium without glands. The normal thick white vaginal secretion is acid (pH 5). In response to oestrogens the stratified cells accumulate glycogen, which is converted to lactic acid by Döderlein's bacilli, which are constantly present. Vaginal infection occurs more easily when the acidity is lowered or absent before puberty or after the menopause.

Infection with *Trichomonas vaginalis*

This organism is a protozoon, about the size of a leucocyte, which is actively motile by means of its flagella (Fig. 16.1). It causes a profuse yellow purulent discharge, often containing tiny bubbles. There may be minute red erosions over the cervix and vaginal fornices, and severe secondary vulvitis. The infection is usually transmitted by intercourse, but occasionally by indirect contact. The organism is detected by placing a little of the discharge in a drop of normal saline on a slide and searching for the motile organisms with a microscope.

Trichomoniasis is treated with metronidazole (Flagyl). A single dose of 2 g orally is often effective, but this may well be followed by 1 g daily for 7 days. Recurrences are usually

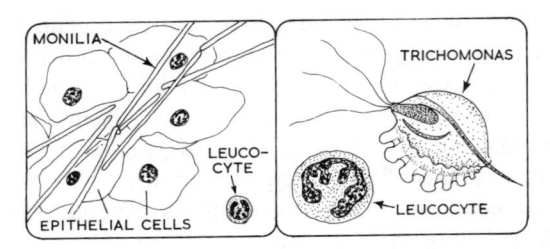

Fig. 16.1 Microscopic appearances of *Monilia* and *Trichomonas*. The latter is shown at a higher magnification.

caused by reinfection, so the sexual partner is given the same treatment.

Infection with *Candida albicans*

This occurs most frequently during pregnancy, or with diabetic glycosuria, but may occur at any time. White patches are seen on the vaginal surface or vulva, and in pregnancy the vagina may be filled with semisolid masses of mycelium. The mycelial threads of the organism are seen in films of the discharge (Fig. 16.1). It is usually, but not always, conveyed sexually. For treatment see p. 242.

Infection with *Gardnerella vaginalis*

This organism is a small Gram-negative bacillus which causes an offensive greyish-white discharge. Microscopical examination shows vaginal cells stippled with adherent bacteria. The treatment is similar to that for trichomoniasis.

Vulvo-vaginitis of children

In the absence of vaginal acidity infection with coliforms and other organisms may occur, especially if there is a lack of hygiene, or a vaginal foreign body is present. Trichomonads or gonococci are occasionally found, and may be an indication of sexual abuse by an adult.

There is profuse yellow discharge with vulvitis and local irritation. The cause must be found and treated, but oestrogens will assist by inducing the development of a more resistant adult type of epithelium. Ethinyl oestradiol 10 micrograms daily by mouth may be given with local application of dinoestrol cream through a small tube.

Atrophic vaginitis

This is a non-specific infection caused by organisms that gain a foothold after the menopause in the absence of the acid barrier. It may spread upward to the endometrium (p. 251). There is thin purulent discharge, sometimes blood-stained. Vaginal stenosis may be a sequel. For treatment oestrogens may be applied locally as dinoestrol cream through a tubular applicator. Ethinyl oestradiol 50 micrograms daily can also be given systemically, with douches of lactic acid 2%.

Vaginitis secondary to other conditions

Vaginitis will occur (1) with any retained foreign body such as a pessary or tampon, (2) with irritant douche fluid or chemical pessaries, (3) with vesical or rectal fistulae, and (4) with foul discharge from a neoplasm.

CERVICITIS AND ENDOMETRITIS
Pathways of infection

Normally there are no bacteria in the uterine cavity. Any endometrial infection tends to die out after a few menstrual cycles, but infection often persists in the deep cervical glands.

More than one type of organism may be found, and then relatively innocuous bacteria may become pathogenic. The following types of infection occur:

1. Acute ascending uterine infection may follow abortion or labour, and is caused by a variety of organisms, including streptococci, coliforms and staphylococci.
2. Gonococci may infect the cervix, and the infection may ascend through the uterus to the tubes.
3. Chlamydia may infect the cervix and also the tubes.
4. Endometritis may occur after the menopause from ascending infection when the vaginal acidity falls.
5. Malignant neoplasms of the cervix or endometrium may become necrotic and infected.
6. Human papillomavirus (HPV) may infect the cervical squamous epithelium, and is under suspicion as a cause of some cases of cervical cancer.
7. Tuberculous endometritis differs from the conditions already listed in that it is caused by descending infection from primary lesions in the tubes.

Cervicitis

In *acute cervicitis*, whether puerperal or gonococcal, there is profuse purulent discharge from the cervical canal.

The term *chronic cervicitis* is ill-defined and over-used. Round cell infiltration can be found in the wall of the cervix of many parous women, but for practical usage the term might be restricted to cases with persistent mucopurulent discharge from the cervical canal. The cervix is often patulous, and may be fixed by paracervical fibrosis. The cervical mucosa is hypertrophic, sometimes forming small polypoid tags at the external os. The bacterial flora is very mixed. For treatment see p. 250.

Various cervical lesions

These are placed here for convenience, although they are not of infective origin.

Nabothian cysts

Cervical glands may become distended with opaque mucus and project on the vaginal surface of the cervix. Such cysts are of no importance.

Cervical ectropion

If the cervix is badly torn the endocervical columnar epithelium is exposed, and there is often a mucoid discharge. A torn cervix may be incompetent during pregnancy.

Cervical erosion

This is a bad term, as an erosion is not an ulcer. It is sometimes associated with chronic cervicitis, but it is not itself an inflammatory lesion. A red velvety zone is seen around the external os, where the pink stratified epithelium has been replaced by an outgrowth of columnar epithelium from cervical glands. The surface may be smooth or papillary.

Erosions are common in normal pregnancy and in patients taking oral contraceptives, and are thought to be caused by the action of oestrogens. After pregnancy or on stopping the pill they often, but not invariably, resolve. Erosions may also occur without evident cause.

Erosions may also (uncommonly) occur in children as 'congenital erosions', presumably because the upgrowth of stratified epithelium has not reached the external os.

Many erosions cause no symptoms and need no treatment, but there may be a blood-stained mucoid discharge, or post-coital bleeding. Erosions have no relation to cervical dysplasia and carcinoma.

Treatment of cervical discharge

Having excluded cervical cancer by examination of cervical smears and, should the smears prove to be abnormal, by colposcopy and biopsy, excessive cervical secretion can be reduced by:

1. Using the hot wire or diathermy cautery to lay open infected glands and coagulate the superficial epithelium of the cervical canal and over an erosion. This is best done with an anaesthetic, though it is possible without. Discharge increases for about seven days until sloughs separate and the superficial epithelium regenerates from the deeper parts of the glands. Secondary haemorrhage occasionally occurs, but can be controlled by vaginal packing. Stenosis is an uncommon sequel of cauterization.
2. Alternatively the tissues can be destroyed by freezing with a cryoprobe, which produces intense cold by rapid vaporization of liquefied gas. This can be done without anaesthesia.
3. A CO_2 laser beam may be used.
4. Amputation of the cervix is unsatisfactory, as only part of the infected cervix is removed, and abortion may occur in a subsequent pregnancy.
5. If there is associated uterine or tubal disease in parous women, total hysterectomy is recommended.

Acute endometritis

May be puerperal, or a transitory event in gonorrhoea.

Uterine tuberculosis

This recurs in association with tubal infection. Tubercles are found in the endometrium, and there is often excessive or irregular menstrual loss. For diagnosis and treatment see p. 257.

Atrophic endometritis

Ascending infection with coliforms and streptococci may occur when the vaginal acidity falls after menopause. The uterus becomes lined with granulation tissue, and if the cervical canal is blocked the body of the uterus becomes distended with pus (*pyometra*). Atrophic endometritis causes a thin bloodstained purulent discharge; but if pyometra supervenes there will be pelvic discomfort, and gradual enlargement of the uterus. Fever is surprisingly uncommon.

Pyometra may also be caused by blockage of the cervix by carcinoma, or from stenosis after radiotherapy.

Treatment

The cervix is dilated, and the uterus is gently curetted to exclude carcinoma, taking care not to perforate the thin wall. A catheter is introduced to allow drainage and the instillation of acriflavine in glycerine, and ethinyl oestradiol 50 micrograms daily is given by mouth. Pyometra may recur, when hysterectomy is required.

SALPINGO-OÖPHORITIS

Aetiology

1. Infection of the tubes and ovaries may follow delivery or abortion, when *Streptococci* ascend from the placental site or from a cervical laceration by the lymphatics or the

cellular spaces. Puerperal infection by other organisms less commonly damages the tubes.
2. *Gonococci* may ascend by the uterine lumen from a primary cervicitis.
3. *Chlamydial infection* of the cervix, which may there cause no noticeable symptoms, may subsequently ascend to the tubes.
4. *Tuberculous* salpingitis may be due to blood spread from a distant focus.
5. Any pelvic infection, such as appendicitis or an infected ovarian cyst, may secondarily involve the tube.
6. Salpingitis may occasionally follow insertion of an intrauterine contraceptive device.

Pathology

Gonococcal salpingitis is usually acute in onset, streptococcal salpingitis may be acute or insidious, and chlamydial or tuberculous salpingitis is chronic.

In *acute salpingitis*, the tube is congested and oedematous. Pus escapes from the abdominal ostium, and in the streptococcal cases organisms also spread directly through the wall to cause pelvic peritonitis. Resolution may occur at this stage, but often swelling of the mucosa and adherence of its folds blocks the ends of the tube so that it becomes distended with pus, forming a thick-walled and retort-shaped *pyosalpinx* (Fig. 16.2). Less active infection causes a *hydrosalpinx*, when the tube is equally distended, but with thin walls and clear fluid. The contents of a hydrosalpinx or long-standing pyosalpinx are usually sterile, but secondary infection with coliforms or other organisms may occur and cause an acute exacerbation. Salpingitis may also cause tubal blockage with thickened walls, but without distention (*interstitial salpingitis*).

The ovary is usually involved, and is often buried in adhesions and contains follicular cysts. Sometimes an infected

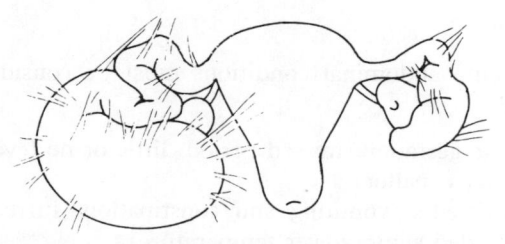

Fig. 16.2 Bilateral salpingo-oöphoritis, with blocked and distended tubes.

tube comes to communicate with a small ovarian cyst to form a *tubo-ovarian cyst or abscess*. Salpingo-oöphoritis is nearly always bilateral, and the dense adhesions formed may hold the uterus in retroversion. Salpingitis is often 'polymicrobial'.

Acute salpingitis

Symptoms and signs

In gonorrhoea upward spread to the tubes is often deferred until the succeeding menstrual period. Puerperal salpingitis is part of widespread pelvic inflammation, and often only recognized after some days of a febrile puerperium.

Severe symptoms arise when the peritoneum is involved. There is sharp lower abdominal pain, usually bilateral. The menstrual rhythm is often upset, and a profuse period occurs. There is muco-purulent discharge from associated cervicitis. Much vomiting or any prolonged change in bowel habit is unusual.

On examination there is fever (39°C+) and lower abdominal tenderness and resistance. There is extreme tenderness in both lateral vaginal fornices, which usually prevents precise examination, but inflammatory masses consisting of the matted tubes and adjacent structures may be felt.

Diagnosis

Other acute abdominal conditions must be considered, but especially:

1. Ectopic gestation (missed period, little or no fever, unilateral signs, pallor).
2. Appendicitis (vomiting and constipation, furred tongue, right-sided signs, lower temperature).
3. Torsion of an ovarian cyst (well-defined lump).

Treatment

Rest in bed. Because no single antibiotic is effective against the known pathogens in salpingitis a two day regime is recommended, e.g. Ampicillin plus metronidazole (Flagyl). Most cases respond to conservative treatment, and laparotomy is only required for cases in which the diagnosis is doubtful, or cases that fail to improve after some days. Spreading peritonitis seldom occurs, so that conservative treatment is usually possible in the initial stage.

Chronic salpingitis

Symptoms and signs

Chronic salpingitis may follow an acute attack, or may have an insidious onset. Recurrent subacute attacks may occur, or there may be persistent pelvic pain and backache. Congestive premenstrual dysmenorrhoea occurs, and sometimes dyspareunia. There is often menorrhagia. Associated cervicitis causes muco-purulent discharge. Tubal blockage causes sterility. There may be no fever except in an exacerbation. The uterus may be held in retroversion with fixed tender tubo-ovarian masses behind it, commonly bilateral, but of unequal size.

Diagnosis

Cases of ovarian endometriosis may be indistinguishable, with pain, sterility, menorrhagia and similar signs; except that there is no cervicitis. A hydrosalpinx may be mistaken for an ovarian cyst until the abdomen is opened. Laparoscopy may sometimes be helpful, but if there is a definite swelling laparotomy will be required in any case.

Treatment

1. Conservative treatment consists of antibiotics during exacerbations. A two day regime is best.
2. Laparotomy is recommended if there are recurrent acute attacks, if there are persistent symptoms that fail to respond to conservative treatment, or if there is a large pelvic mass. Infected tissue is excised, and as the cervix is often infected total hysterectomy is often wise; it is sometimes possible to conserve ovarian tissue. A pelvic abscess may be drained vaginally.
3. In a few cases salpingostomy or other plastic operations may be attempted for sterility due to blocked tubes, but success is infrequent because the ciliated epithelium has often been irretrievably damaged.

Tuberculous salpingitis

See p. 257.

Oöphoritis

Inflammation of the ovary accompanies salpingitis and is due to the same causes. Other pelvic infections such as appendicitis may involve the ovary, and an ovarian cyst that becomes twisted or otherwise damaged may become infected. Oöphoritis sometimes occurs in mumps.

The ovary may contain single or multiple abscesses, or a tubo-ovarian abscess may occur (see p. 253). The ovary may be buried in dense adhesions which cause sterility. Loculated collections of fluid in these adhesions may mimic ovarian cysts clinically. Excessive and frequent menstruation occurs.

The diagnosis and treatment are similar to those for salpingitis.

PELVIC PERITONITIS AND CELLULITIS

Pelvic peritonitis

Pelvic peritonitis may be caused by appendicitis, diverticulitis or infection of a carcinoma of the bowel. Gynaecological causes include:

1. Puerperal or postabortal infection.
2. Gonococcal infection.
3. Pelvic tuberculosis.
4. Infection of an ovarian cyst.
5. Infection of a uterine neoplasm.
6. Infected haematoma, after an operation or ectopic pregnancy.

In peritonitis an effusion occurs, which may be absorbed, become encysted, or become an abscess. Subsequent adhesions may cause sterility and bind the uterus in retroversion.

The history varies with the cause. In acute cases there is severe lower abdominal pain, with vomiting and fever. The lower abdomen is tender and rigid, and there is tenderness and fullness in the vaginal fornices. If an abscess forms the temperature swings, the mass becomes more definite, then softens, and if left may point rectally or above the inguinal ligament.

Treatment varies with the cause. Most gynaecological cases are localized and should be treated conservatively by rest and chemotherapy unless an abscess forms. A pelvic abscess can sometimes be drained through the posterior fornix.

Pelvic cellulitis (parametritis)

Pelvic cellulitis and peritonitis are usually combined in varying degree. Infection of pelvic cellular tissue may follow abortion or delivery, or gynaecological operations or irradiation of infected neoplasms.

The main features are pelvic discomfort, persistent fever, and an indurated mass in one or both fornices with fixation of the cervix. Slow but complete resolution usually occurs, although an abscess may form. Sometimes fibrosis persists and fixes the cervix to one side. Antibiotics are used if the causal organism is susceptible. An abscess requires drainage.

PELVIC TUBERCULOSIS

Pathology

Tubercle bacilli are thought to reach the female genital organs by the blood stream from a distant focus, although the primary focus is not always evident. The bacilli are usually of the human type. Infection of the pelvic organs occurs in cases of tuberculous peritonitis; conversely the pelvic organs may be the initial source of peritoneal infection. The tubes are the commonest site of the disease, and ovarian and uterine infections are fairly common. Infections of the cervix, vagina and vulva are very rare and arise from descending infection.

A tuberculous pyosalpinx is retort-shaped and usually bilateral, contains caseous pus, and has tubercles on the peritoneal surface. Ovarian abscesses may occur. In the uterus tubercles are found in both muscle and endometrium. In the cervix, vagina and vulva ulcers very rarely occur.

Symptoms and signs

Pelvic tuberculosis occurs most frequently in young adults. In Britain today many cases are discovered only during investigation of infertility or menorrhagia. Histological examination of curettings may reveal tubercles, and the bacilli can be grown in cultures made from fresh (unfixed) curettings. If the uterine tubes are found to be blocked with no evidence of any other type of infection tuberculosis should be considered. A few cases are discovered only at laparoscopy or laparotomy, when tubercles are seen on the peritoneal surfaces.

Apart from infertility there may be no symptoms, but in more active cases there may be pelvic pain and dysmenorrhoea, sometimes with acute attacks caused by secondary infection with other organisms. Menorrhagia may occur, although amenorrhoea occurs in advanced cases.

If there are physical signs they are those of chronic salpingitis. Ascites sometimes occurs, when tapping yields blood-stained fluid. In about one-fifth of cases X-ray examination of the chest shows active, or recently active, lesions. In females coincidental infection of the urinary tract is uncommon. Advanced cases, now seldom seen, become cachectic, with fever, diarrhoea and vomiting.

Treatment

Any treatment required for pulmonary disease would be the first consideration, but for pelvic disease typical treatment would be rifampicin 600 mg and isoniazid 300 mg by mouth daily. Ethambutol might be used in an acute stage, but not long continued because of its toxicity. Endometrial biopsy is repeated at 6-monthly intervals, and chemotherapy is discontinued only when there has been no evidence of activity for a year.

Surgical treatment is advised only for cases with symptoms or localized masses which do not respond to chemotherapy, when hysterectomy and bilateral salpingo-oöphorectomy is usually required. Sometimes the diagnosis is made only on opening the abdomen for ascites or chronic salpingitis, and then diseased organs are removed if this can be easily done; but it is dangerous to attempt to free widespread adhesions to bowel.

17

Tumours

TUMOURS OF THE VULVA, URETHRA AND VAGINA

Vulval tumours

Benign tumours

Fibromata and *lipomata* are often pedunculated and are easily excised. *Condylomata acuminata*, which often appear as small papillomatous warts, are usually inflammatory rather than neoplastic, and are caused by infection with human papilloma virus (HPV). Such condylomata can be excised with diathermy or treated by cryosurgery or with a laser. *Hidradenoma* is a rare benign solid tumour that arises from sweat glands. *Pigmented moles* occasionally give rise to *melanomata*; if there is any suspicion they should be widely excised; minor inadequate surgery is dangerous. *Endometriomata* may occur.

Epithelioma of the vulva

Pathology. Vulval carcinoma occurs most frequently in elderly women and often follows leukoplakia. It is a squamous-celled growth, with the rare exception of adenocarcinoma arising in Bartholin's gland. The growth most frequently starts on the labium majus, but also occurs on the clitoris, labia minora or near the urethra. When first seen the growth is usually ulcerated, but papillary and nodular types occur, and growth may also begin in a deep leukoplakic fissure. The inguinal lymphatic glands are soon involved, with subsequent spread to the gland of Cloquet in the femoral canal and thence to the iliac glands.

Symptoms. There is often long-standing pruritus from leukoplakia. A nodule appears which breaks down to form an ulcer with everted edges, and there is bloodstained discharge. Pain is due to secondary sepsis, or to involvement of deep structures. The inguinal glands are enlarged by metastases or sepsis.

Treatment. In operable cases the whole vulva is excised with bilateral dissection of the inguinal, femoral and iliac glands. Radical surgery gives much better results than radiotherapy, although this may be used for recurrences.

Malignant melanoma

Malignant melanoma is rare. When possible, the vulva and pigmented tumour is excised with the lymphatic glands, but the prognosis is very bad.

Other vulval swellings

Varicosities of vulval veins first appear during pregnancy, but may persist afterwards, and can then be treated by excision.

A *Bartholin cyst* is caused by blockage of the duct of the vestibular gland, and the translucent cyst contains mucoid fluid. It is treated by incision and suturing its lining to the skin (marsupialization). A cyst may become infected.

Urethral swellings

Although some of these are not neoplastic it is convenient to describe them here.

Urethral caruncle

A caruncle appears at the posterior lip of the urethral orifice as a small red pedunculated swelling, sometimes very tender (Fig. 17.1). There may be pain on micturition and dyspareunia, with slight bleeding.

Caruncles consist of granulation tissue, or of what appears to be vascular adenomatous tissue. Both types are due to tissue proliferation in response to local infection. The adenomatous element arises from glands in the floor of the urethra.

Treatment. Excision. Any urinary infection must be dealt with. Caruncles often recur but are not malignant.

Prolapse of the urethral mucosa

To be distinguished from a caruncle. The swelling involves the whole circumference of the orifice. If causing discomfort the redundant mucosa is excised.

Urethral diverticulum

Although this is not rare it is often overlooked. There may be a fluctuant swelling under the anterior vaginal wall, and if the diverticulum becomes infected there is dysuria with intermittent discharge of pus. Diagnosis is made by ureth-

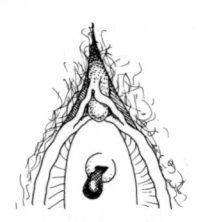

Fig. 17.1 Urethral caruncle.

roscopy and radiological examination after filling the urethra with radio-opaque fluid. If there are symptoms the diverticulum is excised.

Carcinoma of the urethra

Very rare. Both squamous-cell carcinoma and adenocarcinoma occur. If low down the treatment is as for vulval carcinoma; if high up radical urethrocystectomy is required.

Vaginal tumours

Primary carcinoma

A rare tumour of the elderly, that resembles carcinoma of the cervix, with ulceration and bleeding. Treated by local application of caesium.

A few cases of carcinoma of the vagina have occurred in teenage girls whose mothers were treated with stilboestrol during pregnancy. Vaginal adenosis, with columnar gland formation in the vaginal vault, usually precedes the carcinoma. Other oestrogens have not been incriminated. If there is such a risk the girl must be examined regularly with the speculum, vaginal cytology and the colposcope.

Secondary carcinoma

Secondary carcinoma may follow uterine carcinoma. There may be direct spread from the cervix, or metastasis from carcinoma of the body of the uterus, sometimes as an isolated suburethral nodule. Vaginal recurrence after hysterectomy for cancer may occur, and is treated by radiotherapy.

Secondary choriocarcinoma

This occurs as a purple vascular tumour (p. 68).

Endometrioma of the recto-vaginal septum

(See p. 298).

Gaertner's cyst

(See p. 219).

TUMOURS OF THE UTERUS

Benign tumours

Fibromyomata

Pathology. Fibromyomata are the commonest of all uterine tumours. They are seldom found before the age of 30, and never develop for the first time after the menopause. They are more common in nulliparae.

Fibroids occur 15 times more often in the body of the uterus than in the cervix. Seedlings first appear in the uterine wall, and grow slowly, compressing the surrounding tissue to form a capsule. The tumours are gradually extruded from

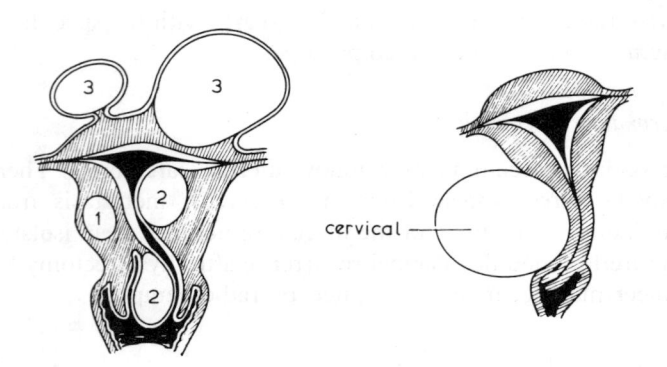

Fig. 17.2 Fibromyomata: (1) interstitial, (2) subendometrial, (3) subperitoneal.

their initial *interstitial* position towards the uterine cavity to become *subendometrial*, or towards the peritoneal surface to become *subperitoneal*; and in either case may become pedunculated. Fibromyomata are often multiple, and may grow to enormous size (Fig. 17.2).

Fibroids are benign. Small tumours consist of smooth muscle fibres (myomata) but large tumours also contain fibrous tissue (fibromyomata). They are whiter in colour than the surrounding muscle, and their whorled structure can be seen with the naked eye. The tumours tend to outgrow their blood supply and then to show degenerative changes, although enormous hypertrophy of the uterine vessels occurs.

Fibromyomata may distort or displace the uterus, pushing it into retroversion, or to one side.

1. Subendometrial tumours first project into the uterine cavity so that the endometrial area is enlarged; and may then become pedunculated, when the uterus contracts to expel the polyp through the dilated cervix. Rarely chronic uterine inversion may follow.
2. Interstitial fibromyomata also distort the uterine cavity and increase the endometrial area.
3. Subperitoneal tumours are often pedunculated.
4. Cervical fibromyomata may greatly elongate the cervical canal and displace the body of the uterus upwards. They may also grow between the layers of the broad ligament, sometimes displacing or compressing the ureter.

In many cases not only is the uterine cavity enlarged, but the endometrium is hypertrophic, and the uterine muscle may show diffuse hyperplasia. The ovaries often contain follicular cysts.

Aetiology. The aetiology of fibromyomata is obscure. On the inconstant evidence of the changes in the ovaries and the endometrium it is suggested that fibroids represent an abnormal response to oestrogens, although it is not known why the reaction is localized to certain parts of the muscle. These tumours are very common in negresses.

Secondary changes. These are as follows:

1. Degenerative changes are common because fibromyomata tend to overgrow their blood supply. *Atrophy*, which is seldom more than partial, occurs after the menopause. *Hyaline degeneration* is common in large or pedunculated tumours, and is without clinical significance. Both connective tissue and muscle fibres are involved. *Fatty degeneration* particularly involves the muscle fibres, and proceeds to *calcareous degeneration*, when the fat breaks down to soaps that take up calcium salts. This change is most common after the menopause. X-ray examination will show calcification. *Red degeneration* is due to a relatively acute interference with blood supply, and is usually but not invariably seen during pregnancy. Possibly the rapid growth of the uterus kinks the capsular vessels: at any rate these vessels are often thrombosed. The tumour swells, softens, and becomes pinkish-red in colour. On microscopical examination a few surviving fibres are seen lying among dead fibres. Fever, pain and vomiting occur. *Cystic degeneration* follows hyaline or red degeneration, and irregular cavities containing serous fluid appear.
2. *Torsion* of a pedunculated fibromyoma, or a whole tumour mass with the uterus, is a rare complication which causes acute pain, shock and vomiting. The tumour may become necrotic from loss of blood supply, or the tumour may acquire a 'parasitic' blood supply from omental adhesions.
3. *Infection.* The capsule of a submucous fibroid may be damaged, when infection can occur and the necrotic tumour is slowly extruded.
4. *Impaction.* A tumour that fills the pelvis and displaces the bladder (especially a cervical tumour) may cause urinary retention. This usually occurs at a menstrual period or

during pregnancy, but may also occur after the menopause when an abdominal tumour shrinks and suddenly sinks into the pelvis. Bowel symptoms are surprisingly uncommon with pelvic fibromyomata.

5. *Malignant change.* Sarcomatous change occurs in less than 0.2% of fibromyomata. The change is most common in large tumours. There is rapid enlargement, with pain, ascites and sometimes irregular or postmenopausal bleeding.
6. *Fibromyomata and pregnancy.* Fibromyomata may cause sterility or abortion; or obstructed labour if situated in the lower uterine segment. Red degeneration, torsion and impaction are more frequent in pregnancy, and a tumour is sometimes damaged and infected during labour.

Symptoms. Many fibromyomata do not cause symptoms and do not require treatment. The commonest symptom is *menorrhagia*, caused by endometrial hyperplasia or enlargement of the endometrial surface, or interference with uterine contractions. Menstrual loss is increased and prolonged, and the cycle is eventually shortened; severe anaemia may result. Postmenopausal bleeding does not occur unless the tumour is extruded as a polyp, or becomes sarcomatous. *Pain* is unusual with uncomplicated tumours, but uterine colic may occur during the expulsion of a polyp. Pain occurs with the following complications: red degeneration, torsion, infection, sarcomatous change. With impaction painful *retention* occurs. (Pain associated with fibroids is often due to coincidental endometriosis.) Concern about a palpable *abdominal tumour* is sometimes the only complaint.

Signs. Large tumours are felt on abdominal examination as hard painless tumours which rise up out of the pelvis. The tumour may be single and rounded, or consist of a group of rounded bosses. It is dull to percussion and no free fluid is evident. On auscultation a uterine souffle may be heard, as a result of the rich flow through the uterine vessels. On pelvic examination, the cervix is found to be attached to the tumour mass.

Smaller tumours are found on pelvic examination as hard painless tumours attached to the uterus, though a pedunculated soft fibromyoma may simulate an ovarian tumour. A solitary interstitial fibromyoma is difficult to recognize as the uterine outline is smooth, although enlarged.

Diagnosis. An interstitial tumour with degenerative softening may be difficult to distinguish from the pregnant uterus, but there is no amenorrhoea, nor is there cervical softening. Fibromyomata and pregnancy may co-exist, and in difficult cases a pregnancy test is required. Ultrasonic examination is useful.

Ovarian tumours are usually cystic, but a solid tumour may be mistaken for a pedunculated fibromyoma.

In cases of tumours with postmenopausal bleeding the possibility of uterine cancer (especially of the body of the uterus) must be considered, and this is far more common than sarcomatous change in a fibromyoma.

Inflammatory masses and endometriosis may cause bleeding, but are tender, and less well defined than fibromyomata.

Treatment. Small symptomless tumours do not require treatment, but large tumours nearly always need to be removed. Treatment is urgently required for retention of urine or torsion, is essential for menorrhagia or suspected sarcoma, and is sometimes required for pain or sterility. The symptoms of red degeneration usually resolve with rest, though the pain may be severe enough to need morphia for relief.

At present most cases are treated surgically. Abdominal hysterectomy, with conservation of the ovaries, is performed in the majority of cases, but abdominal myomectomy is chosen whenever possible in nulliparae under 40, or in parous women who hope for further children. Myomectomy is more difficult then hysterectomy, and the fibromyomata may recur. Solitary polypoid tumours may be removed by vaginal myomectomy.

Menorrhagia caused by small fibromyomata, whose presence is confirmed by ultrasound, may sometimes be controlled by prostaglandin synthetase inhibitors such as mefenamic acid 500 mg thrice daily. Danazol, or synthetic analogues of GnRH, which inhibit pituitary secretion of gonadotrophins and therefore ovarian oestrogen production, are more likely to be effective.

Adenomyoma

See endometriosis, p. 298.

Endometrial polypi

Pathology. These are adenomata. They occur most commonly near the menopause, but are seen in both younger and older women. Usually they arise near the internal tubal orifice, as soft pink tumours less than 1 cm in diameter (Fig. 17.3). They have a covering of endometrium, although squamous metaplasia often occurs. There is an oedematous stroma, in which endometrial glands lie, some of which are cystic, and many of which show incomplete response to the ovarian hormones. Malignant change is rare, but occasionally occurs.

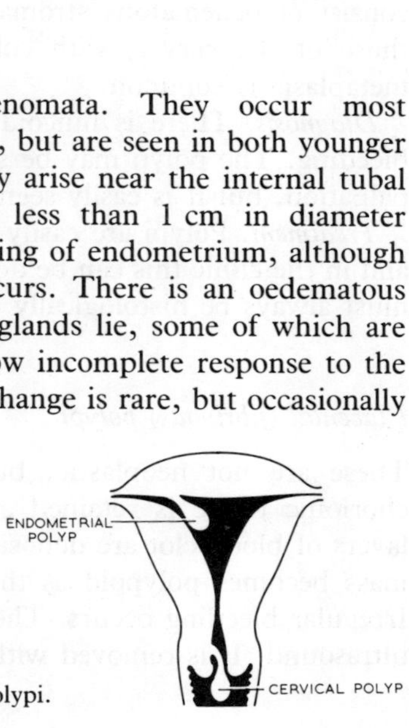

Fig. 17.3 Uterine adenomyomatous polypi.

Clinical features. Small polypi may cause no symptoms, but those more than 5 mm in diameter usually cause menorrhagia or irregular bleeding, and sometimes mucoid discharge. Uterine colic or uterine enlargement does not occur. Diagnosis may be made by hysteroscopy, if available, otherwise with the curette or uterine forceps after dilating the cervix.

Treatment. The polyp is curetted away. Histological examination is always prudent.

Cervical polypi

Pathology. Some are solitary adenomata, but many of them are not true neoplasms, but are the result of proliferation of the endocervical epithelium in response to infection to oestrogens. Small soft pink polypi appear at the external os. They consist of oedematous stroma containing glands resembling those of the cervix, with columnar epithelium. Squamous metaplasia is common.

Diagnosis. There is mucoid discharge and slight irregular bleeding. The polyp may be so soft that it is not noticed on palpation, but it is easily seen with a speculum.

Treatment. Polypi are easily removed by twisting them off, and in the clinic this can be done without pain, but the polyp must always be histologically examined.

Placental (fibrinous) polypi

These are not neoplastic, but occur when a fragment of chorionic tissue is retained after abortion or delivery, and layers of blood clot are deposited on the retained tissue. The mass becomes polypoid as the uterus contracts to expel it. Irregular bleeding occurs. The polyp can be recognized with ultrasound. It is removed with uterine forceps.

Malignant tumours

Carcinoma of the cervix

Aetiological factors. The commonest age at which cervical cancer appears is between 40 and 50, but many cases are seen in older and younger women. About 95% of the patients are parous. The incidence is increased in women of low socio-economic status, and in some parts of Africa, Asia and South America. There is much to suggest that the causative factor is transmitted by coitus. It is almost unknown in virgins. Aggressive cancer can occur in young women who are sexually active, and in women with many sexual partners. It is uncommon in Jewesses; although it has been suggested that this is because of male circumcision, less irregular sexual experience is a more likely explanation.

The virus of herpes genitalis has been found in some cases, but the association is inconstant, and the virus is not thought to cause the growth. More suspicion is now directed towards human papilloma virus (HPV).

A pre-invasive stage (*carcinoma in situ*) of several years duration precedes the development of many cases of invasive cancer. Pre-invasive cancer does not cause symptoms and can only be discovered by careful examination of vaginal smears and colposcopy (p. 273), and when necessary, biopsy. A proportion of the cases, perhaps 20% over 10 years, eventually progress to become invasive.

Pathology. The growth usually arises near the squamo-columnar junction on the portio vaginalis, but sometimes arises from the epithelium of the cervical canal or glands. The growth infiltrates into the cervix, and also may project from the surface. Either of these processes may predominate. When the growth outgrows its blood supply, necrosis and secondary infection follow, with bleeding and foul discharge. The friable growth breaks away to leave an ulcer crater, which progressively extends. Endocervical carcinoma grows in the canal and first expands the cervix, but subsequent spread is in the same manner. Cervical carcinoma extends by:

1. *Local spread*. The growth invades the adjacent vaginal vault. Lateral spread into the broad ligament fixes the cervix, and in later stages may obstruct the ureter. Anterior spread reaches the bladder, and in late stages necrosis may cause a vesicovaginal fistula. Posterior spread involves the uterosacral ligaments, and later the rectum, and may cause a rectovaginal fistula. Upward spread is often limited, but obstruction to the cervical canal may cause a pyometra.
2. *Lymphatic spread* occurs to the iliac glands on the pelvic side wall and obturator fossa, and also backwards to the sacral glands.
3. *Blood spread* causes distant metastases, but is not common until late in the disease. Osseous, cerebral and pulmonary lesions are commonest.

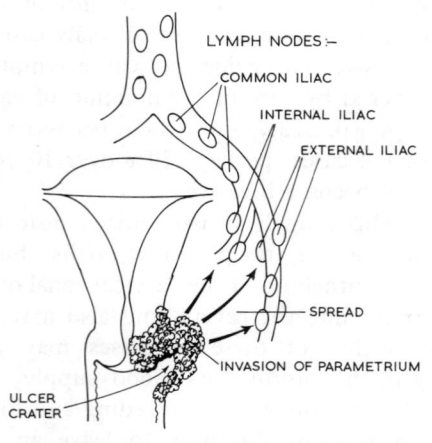

Fig. 17.4 Diagram to show deep infiltration and lymphatic spread of carcinoma of cervix.

4. *Vaginal implantation* may occur, but lymphatic spread may equally explain the isolated vaginal metastases that are occasionally seen.

Histology. Ninety-five per cent of cervical carcinomata arise from squamous cells. This would be expected in growths that arise from the superficial squamous epithelium, but it is also true for growths that start in the cervical canal, probably because the columnar epithelium first undergoes metaplasia. The cells are often undifferentiated, and cell nests are unusual as keratinization does not occur. The most active growths consist of spindle-shaped cells with little resemblance to normal epithelial cells. The remaining 5% of growths are adenocarcinomata.

In carcinoma in situ (pre-invasive carcinoma) the cells resemble those of invasive carcinoma, but there is no evident transgression of the basement membrane.

Vaginal cytology. Early cancer does not cause symptoms, but at this stage exfoliated cancer cells may be recognized in a smear prepared after scraping the cervix with a spatula, or less effectively in secretion aspirated from the posterior fornix. The smear must be fixed immediately, but is stained later in the laboratory, often with Papanicolaou's stain. Malignant cells are large and of bizarre shape, with deeply staining or multiple nuclei showing active mitosis. Routine smears should be taken from all women aged 30 or more, at intervals of less than 3 years. If facilities are available smears might be taken with advantage in younger women and at shorter intervals. Routine examination of 1000 women aged 20 or more will yield about 25 abnormal smears, which urgently require investigation by colposcopy or biopsy. Of these, five are likely to show premalignant change, and one to come from an invasive cancer.

Colposcopy is an outpatient procedure by which the cervix is examined under good illumination with a low-power microscope after application of acetic acid to clarify the cell pattern. Atypical epithelium and aberrant capillary patterns can be recognized, and suspicious areas selected for biopsy.

Cervical biopsy. If any suspicious lesion is seen by naked eye or the colposcope, or if a smear is repeatedly positive, biopsy is essential. Areas which do not stain brown when painted with iodine solution (because the cells do not contain glycogen) are suspicious (Schiller's test). Colposcopy will permit selection of limited areas for bipsy, otherwise the whole squamo-columnar junction is taken with a subjacent cone of tissue that includes most of the cervical canal. A cold knife is used, not diathermy, which might confuse the histological examination.

Histological examination of the cervical tissue may reveal: (1) Metaplasia, in which the cervical columnar cells are replaced by squamous cells. This is a reversible and non-malignant change. (2) Dysplasia, in which there is disordered arrangement and activity of the cells. This may progress to pre-invasive or invasive carcinoma. The international classification of these *cervical intraepithelial neoplastic changes* is:

CIN I: Mild dysplasia, which may regress to metaplasia or progress to CIN II.
CIN II: Moderate dysplasia, which may progress to CIN III.
CIN III: Severe dysplasia, which includes pre-invasive carcinoma (carcinoma in situ).

Symptoms. Once ulceration has occurred there is slight irregular bleeding, especially on examination or intercourse. Diagnosis should be made at this stage, or even earlier by vaginal cytology. Unfortunately cases are often seen when necrosis and infection has caused blood-stained purulent foul discharge, or profuse bleeding. Pain is a late symptom, due to spread of infection, to pyometra, or to extensive spread of growth. With bladder involvement there is frequency, and sometimes haematuria, and finally incontinence if a fistula forms. Uraemia from ureteric obstruction or ascending infection may be the final cause of death. Anaemia and cachexia occur in terminal stages.

Signs. In an early case biopsy is necessary for diagnosis, but cases are still seen in which the diagnosis is dreadfully obvious on clinical examination. Part or the whole of the cervix is replaced by a crater, with friable tissue in the base and edges. The growth is softer than the normal cervix; a probe will sink into it and it bleeds on touching. A cervical erosion may also bleed slightly on touch, but an erosion is firm and not friable. If there is the slightest doubt biopsy is essential.

In a few cases a hypertrophic mass of growth projects ('cauliflower type'). With endocervical carcinoma there may at first be no external evidence of growth, but the cervix is distended to a barrel shape, and friable growth is revealed if the cervix is dilated.

Deep extension of growth into the parametrium may be palpable, especially on rectal examination, which should always be performed.

Stages of cervical carcinoma. An international clinical classification is in use. In brief:

Stage 0:   Pre-invasive carcinoma.
Stage I: Growth confined to the cervix.
Stage IIa: Spread to the vaginal vault, but not below the upper third.
Stage IIb: Spread into the parametrium, but not extending to the pelvic wall.
Stage III: Spread to the lower two-thirds of the vagina, or parametrial spread extending to the pelvic wall.
Stage IV: Metastases outside the pelvis, or involvement of the bladder or rectum.

Prognosis. With treatment the 5-year survival rate for Stage

I growths is more than 75%, for Stage II growths about 50%, and for Stage III and IV growths (together) about 10%.

Treatment of pre-invasive carcinoma. If the tumour has been completely removed by biopsy the case is followed up for life by repeated smears. If lesions are accurately demarcated by colposcopy and biopsy they can be destroyed with a laser. Otherwise the safest course is to remove the uterus with a wide vaginal cuff. The ovaries can be left. This treatment can occasionally be deferred for a time until a pregnancy is achieved or completed.

Treatment of invasive carcinoma. The choice between radiotherapy and surgical treatment for operable cases can be hotly debated. The introduction of new and more powerful sources of radiation has been paralleled by a revival of interest in surgical techniques. Approximately equal results are obtained by the best exponents of the two methods, and the aim must be to select the best treatment for the individual patient, perhaps by combined attack.

Many gynaecologists believe that radiotherapy offers better results than surgery, even for early cases. The immediate risk is very small, and the method can be used for all but the most advanced cases, in which there is a risk of precipitating fistula formation. Radiation from sources placed in the uterus and vagina does not effectively irradiate glands on the pelvic wall, and deep X-ray therapy is therefore directed at these fields.

On the other hand, because a few cases with small primary growths are found to have involved glands, and as there is some doubt whether X-ray treatment will deal effectively with these, some surgeons advise Wertheim's operation (see below) for the early cases.

Method of insertion of caesium or radium. Many different techniques are in use; the following description outlines the Manchester method as an illustration. Under anaesthesia metal tubes holding caesium 137 or radium 226 are placed in a rubber tubular container in the uterine cavity, and in two rubber 'ovoids' which are positioned in the lateral vaginal fornices (Fig. 17.5). The ovoids are designed to hold the element at an appropriate distance from the vaginal wall. The bladder is kept empty with an indwelling catheter. The containers are held in place with an adjustable colpostat or with gauze packing, and their position is checked after insertion by X-ray examination. Two or three separate treatments are given, each lasting between 24 and 36 hours according to the physical calculations, with the object of giving the maximum dose of radiation which will not injure the bladder or rectum. Excessive radiation to the bladder will cause cystitis and occasionally a fistula, and to the rectum will cause proctitis and sometimes stenosis. Vaginal stenosis frequently occurs.

While the sources are being positioned and while they are in place there is a risk to staff and others around the patient. To avoid part of the risk afterloading techniques have been devised. A colpostat with tubes leading to the applications is positioned without haste in the theatre, the patient is transferred to a screened cubicle, and then the sources are quickly introduced.

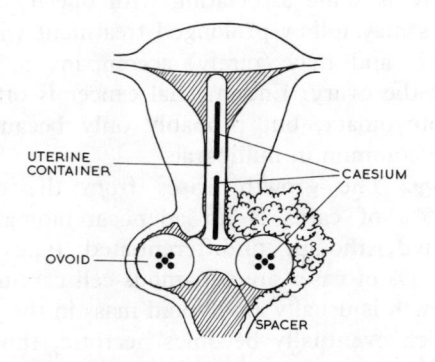

Fig. 17.5 Applications in place for treatment of carcinoma of the cervix with caesium 137.

Wertheim's hysterectomy is a difficult procedure only suitable for fit patients with operable growths (Stages I and IIa). It differs from an ordinary total hysterectomy in the following particulars. The ureter is fully exposed and retracted laterally so that the cardinal ligaments can be divided far out. The uterus, tubes and ovaries, broad ligaments, and upper third of the vagina are removed with as much of the adjacent cellular tissue as possible. Iliac and obturator lymphatic nodes are dissected out. Especial dangers are shock, bleeding from deep veins, and injury to the ureters or bladder.

In advanced cases only palliative treatment is possible, with drugs to relieve pain, although even more extensive operations (*pelvic exenteration*) in which the rectum or bladder is removed with the uterus are occasionally possible. In cases with severe pain intrathecal injection of alcohol to block sensory pathways may be considered.

Endometrial carcinoma

Aetiological factors. This is often but not invariably seen after the menopause. About half of the patients are nulliparous. There is some association with obesity and diabetes. Some cases may follow prolonged treatment with oestrogens (see p. 317) and may (rarely) accompany a granulosa-cell tumour of the ovary. Endometrial cancer is often associated with fibromyomata, but probably only because both conditions are common in nulliparae.

Pathology. The growth arises from the endometrium, and in 95% of cases is an adenocarcinoma, often well-differentiated, though undifferentiated types occur. The remaining 5% of cases are squamous-cell carcinomata.

The growth is usually a polypoid mass in the upper uterine cavity which eventually becomes necrotic, though infection is late because the growth is in a protected situation. In other cases there is less outgrowth, and ulceration predominates.

The growth spreads by:

1. *Local spread*. The muscle wall is infiltrated, and ultimately penetrated; though the thick wall confines the growth for a time. The internal os may be blocked by growth, when pyometra follows.
2. *Lymphatic spread* chiefly follows the ovarian lymphatics to reach the glands around the aorta. In advanced cases the lymphatics around the uterine vessels are also involved, and exceptional spread occurs in lymphatics that accompany the round ligament to reach the inguinal glands. Ovarian metastases are common, by lymphatic pathways.
3. *Blood spread* is not prominent, but widespread metastasis may occur in late stages.
4. *Vaginal implantation* may occur, sometimes low down near the urethra.

Symptoms. Malignant cells may be found by vaginal cytology, but less certainly than with cervical cancer. The first symptom is bloodstained discharge, usually though not invariably occurring after the menopause. Profuse bleeding is less common than with cervical cancer. When infection of the growth occurs the discharge becomes purulent and foul. Slight pain may be due to uterine distention by growth or pyometra, but severe pain is a late event that only occurs when there is extensive spread. Finally, cachexia occurs.

Signs. In most cases the uterus is only slightly enlarged, but in a few it is grossly enlarged by a large florid growth, by a pyometra, or because the growth arises in a fibromyomatous uterus.

Diagnosis depends on diagnostic curettage. Cancer cells may be found in a vaginal smear, but this test does not replace biopsy. Bleeding from atrophic endometritis, an endometrial polyp, or a fibromyomatous polyp can only be distinguished after dilatation of the cervix. A granulosa cell tumour of the ovary will cause postmenopausal bleeding, but the ovarian tumour may be palpable, and the endometrium shows oestrogenic and not neoplastic change. Confusion may also arise when patients have been given oestrogens.

Prognosis. With treatment the 5-year survival rate is over 60%.

Treatment. Ordinary total hysterectomy with bilateral salpingo-oöphorectomy and removal of a wide cuff of vagina gives fairly good results, but a few surgeons advocate Wertheim's hysterectomy, as lymphatic glands are sometimes involved. Radium or caesium is often inserted before operation to reduce the risk of recurrence in the vaginal vault.

This growth is radiosensitive, and if the patient is unfit for operation radium can be used as an alternative, though the results of surgical treatment are better.

Progestogens in large doses (e.g., 17α-hydroxyprogesterone hexanoate 5 g weekly intramuscularly) will cause remission of the growth in some cases. Some surgeons give progestogens both before and after operation.

Stages of endometrial carcinoma. The international clinical classification is:

Stage I: Cancer confined to corpus uteri.
Stage II: Cancer involving both corpus and cervix.
Stage III: Cancer extending beyond the uterus but not outside the pelvis.
Stage IV: Cancer involving the bladder or rectum or extending outside the pelvis.

The classification is of limited value as most cases are placed in Stage I, and the outcome depends far more on the age and general health of the patient and on the depth of invasion of the myometrium.

TUMOURS

Sarcoma of the uterus

Pathology. Uterine sarcoma is an uncommon tumour. Sarcomatous change occurs in less than 0.2% of fibromyomata, and although rare this is yet the commonest type of sarcoma. It is usually a spindle-shaped sarcoma. The histological evidence of malignancy may be doubtful even when the clinical course proves it.

Round-cell sarcoma of the endometrium occurs as a soft large vascular tumour that distends the uterine cavity.

Clinical features. Irregular and heavy uterine bleeding occurs. The tumour grows rapidly, with pain, ascites and cachexia. Diagnosis usually depends on the histological section.

Treatment. The uterus and adnexae are removed, and X-ray therapy may be given. The prognosis is bad.

Mesodermal mixed tumours

Although uncommon, these tumours are less rare than was formerly believed. They arise from the primitive mesoderm from which the Müllerian tract is developed. They are chiefly sarcomatous, but may contain mixed elements, including striped muscle, cartilage or carcinomatous tissue.

In adults the tumour grows as a large fleshy mass in the uterine cavity. A rare variety is the *botryoid (grape-like) sarcoma* of the cervix, usually seen in children. The tumours cause bleeding. They must be removed as radically as possible, but even with additional radiotherapy the prognosis is very bad.

Choriocarcinoma

See p. 68.

TUMOURS OF THE OVARY

Without knowledge of aetiology, with uncertainty about the tissue from which many ovarian tumours arise, and with small distinction between benign and malignant varieties of some tumours, classification of the numerous varieties of ovarian tumours is unsatisfactory. The following list includes all but a few exceedingly rare varieties (see Fig. 17.6):

1. Distention cysts of the follicular apparatus.
    Follicular cysts.
    Lutein cysts.
2. Primary ovarian neoplasms:
    Mucinous cystadenoma and carcinoma.
    Serous (and papilliferous) cystadenoma and carcinoma.
    Endometrioid carcinoma.
    Benign teratoma (dermoid cyst).
    Malignant teratoma.
    Endodermal sinus tumour.
    Brenner tumour.
    Fibroma.
    Granulosa cell tumour.
    Thecoma.
    Androblastoma (arrhenoblastoma).
    Disgerminoma.
3. Metastatic neoplasms.
    Pelvic origin.
    Krukenberg tumour.
4. Endometriosis.

1. Distention cysts of the follicular apparatus

Follicular cysts

These common cysts are often multiple, and are seldom larger than 3 cm in diameter. The cyst wall consists of an incomplete layer of granulosa cells, and outside that the theca layers of the follicle. Follicular cysts do not become malignant, and in most cases are of no clinical significance; but in cystic endometrial hyperplasia (p. 308) the ovary contains follicular cysts with an active layer of granulosa cells.

Lutein cysts

Cystic corpus luteum. The ripe corpus luteum occasionally forms a cyst less than 5 cm in diameter which may be associated with temporary amenorrhoea.

Theca-lutein cyst. Both the granulosa and theca interna cells lining a follicular cyst may become luteinized (without ovulation). The change is most evident in the theca cells, when the term theca-lutein cyst is used. In association with a hydatidiform mole bilateral multilocular theca-lutein cysts may occur, up to 10 cm in diameter, due to the excessive output of chorionic gonadotrophin. A similar change can occur during the induction of ovulation with gonadotrophin, unless the treatment is carefully monitored (p. 325).

Excision of follicular or lutein cysts is not recommended unless the abdomen is opened for some other reason. If seen at laparoscopy they can be punctured with a diathermy needle. Haemorrhage may occur into these cysts, and they should not be mistaken for endometriomata. Occasionally intraperitoneal bleeding from a ruptured follicle or corpus luteum is sufficient to suggest the diagnosis of ectopic pregnancy and require laparotomy.

2. Primary ovarian neoplasm

Mucinous cystadenoma

This is a common ovarian neoplasm. It occurs at any age, though most often between 30 and 60, and may grow to enormous size. The outer wall is smoothly rounded, though rounded bosses may project from it. The cyst contains

1. RETENTION CYSTS

Follicular cysts

Small; often multiple.

Lutein cysts

Often single, but multiple in cases of vesicular mole or with excessive use of gonadotrophins.

2. MUCINOUS CYSTS

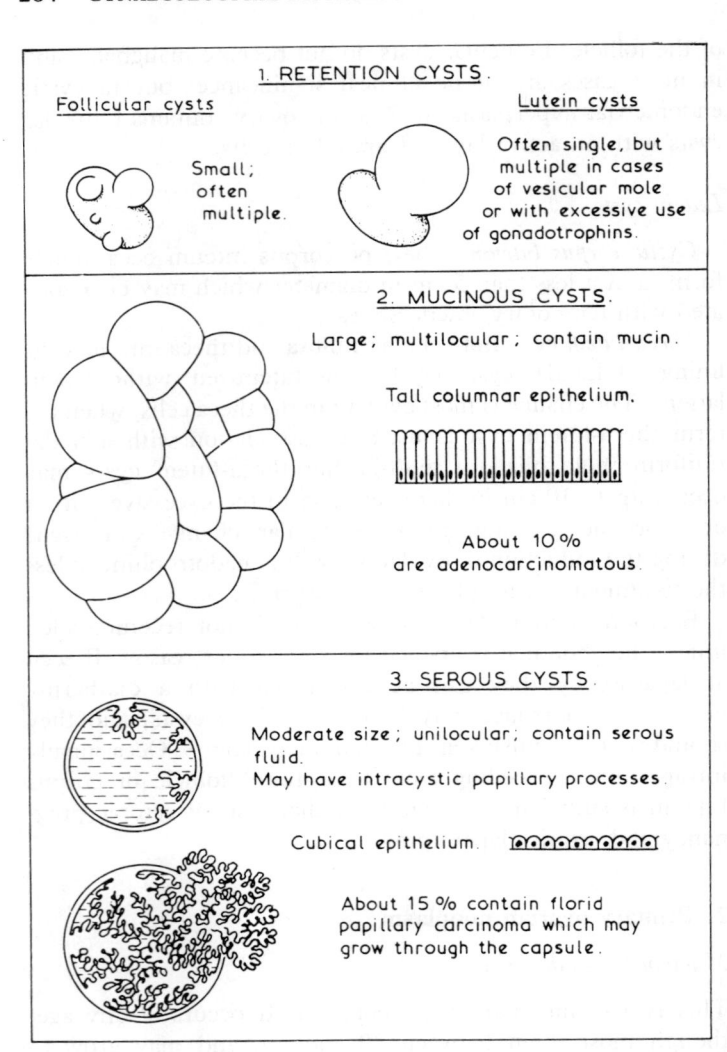

Large; multilocular; contain mucin.

Tall columnar epithelium.

About 10% are adenocarcinomatous.

3. SEROUS CYSTS

Moderate size; unilocular; contain serous fluid.
May have intracystic papillary processes.

Cubical epithelium.

About 15% contain florid papillary carcinoma which may grow through the capsule.

Fig. 17.6 Scheme to show the more common ovarian cysts and tumours.

TUMOURS 285

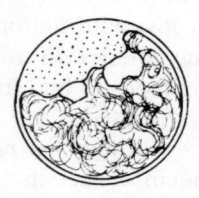

4. TERATOMATOUS CYSTS.

Moderate size; unilocular; with embryonic rudiment containing a mixture of tissues, including teeth.
Cyst contains hair and sebaceous material.
Usually benign.

5. RARE SOLID TERATOMA — highly malignant.

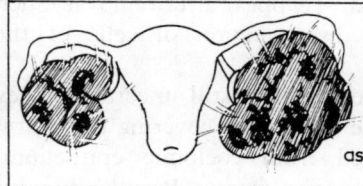

6. ENDOMETRIOMATA.

Bilateral adherent cysts containing altered blood. Secreted by endometriomatous tissue. Nearly always benign but associated with other endometriomata.

7. FIBROMA.
Moderate size; solid; white.
Benign, but may cause ascites.

8. BRENNER TUMOUR.
Resembles fibroma but has epithelial nests among fibrous tissue. Benign.

9. GERM CELL TUMOURS.
Moderate size; solid or partly cystic. Variable appearance and histology. Often malignant.

Granulosa cell tumours and thecomata may secrete oestrogens.
Rare androblastoma secretes androgens.
Disgerminoma resembles seminoma of testis.

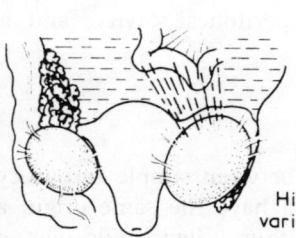

10. MALIGNANT TUMOURS.

May be primary ovarian tumours or metastatic.

Often bilateral, with ascites and fixed to other structures.

Histology depends on origin (some varieties already mentioned above).

Primary endometrioid carcinoma resembles adenocarcinoma of endometrium.

Krukenberg tumour is metastatic from stomach.

multiple loculi full of greenish-yellow slimy mucus. The loculi have a lining of very tall columnar cells, with uniform nuclei situated close to the basement membrane. Fibrous septa separate the loculi, and the epithelium tends to bud into the fibrous tissue and form fresh loculi.

If a mucinous cyst ruptures the condition of *myxoma peritonei* may follow, in which masses of mucin collect in the peritoneal cavity, and repeatedly reappear after removal. Such cases are probably due to dissemination of cells of the tumour.

The origin of these common cysts is still uncertain. They may arise by metaplasia of the epithelium covering the ovary, which was originally derived from coelomic epithelium. Alternatively the tumour may arise from a Brenner tumour (see p. 288). A benign teratoma is sometimes associated with a mucinous tumour.

Mucinous adenocarcinoma

On removal, about 10% of mucinous cysts are found to be malignant. One part of a large tumour may appear malignant and another part benign.

In malignant cysts there is an area of solid white growth, usually adenocarcinoma. The growth infiltrates through the capsule to disseminate in the peritoneal cavity, and also spreads by lymphatics.

Serous (papilliferous) cystadenoma

Distinction is sometimes made between simple serous cysts and papilliferous cysts, but both have the same origin and nature. The *simple serous cyst* is thin-walled, unilocular, and seldom more than 15 cm in diameter. The cyst contains serous fluid and is lined by cubical epithelium. The *papilliferous cyst* is similar except that the lining bears papillary processes that project into the cavity. The papillae may be minute nodules or florid branching processes. Each papilla has a fibrous tissue core and a covering of cubical epithelium. In one-third of cases the cysts are bilateral.

If a benign serous cyst ruptures the fluid is quickly absorbed, but there is a risk of active epithelial fragments becoming implanted.

These tumours probably arise by metaplasia and invagination of the surface epithelium.

Papilliferous carcinoma

About 15% of papilliferous cysts are found to be malignant. In malignant cysts the epithelial layers are several cells deep, and the stroma is invaded. The growth penetrates the cell wall, and then becomes implanted in the peritoneal cavity, causing ascites, often blood-stained.

Clear-cell tumours. These very rare malignant tumours were formerly described as being of mesonephroid origin, with clear cells and projecting nuclei. Probably they are only a variant of papilliferous adenocarcinoma.

Endometrioid carcinoma

Malignant change is very rare in ordinary ovarian endometriosis, but malignant tumours resembling uterine adenocarcinoma may arise primarily in the ovary.

Dermoid cyst (cystic teratoma)

These common cysts are sometimes seen in childhood, but most often during the reproductive period. They grow slowly, are usually less than 10 cm in diameter, and unilateral. At one side of the unilocular cavity is a projection, which is the essential tumour. This 'embryonic rudiment' is covered with skin, bearing hair and sebaceous glands. The greater part of the cyst wall is a fibrous capsule that encloses the yellow sebaceous secretion of these glands. The embryonic rudiment contains a great variety of tissues, chiefly ectodermal such as skin, hair and teeth, and less commonly other tissues such as bone, thyroid, gut, etc.

Dermoid cysts often have a long pedicle, and are especially liable to torsion. Malignant change is rare, but squamous epithelioma may arise.

Teratomata are thought to arise when an unfertilized germ cell divides and proliferates for some unknown reason.

Solid teratoma

These rare highly malignant tumours of young women rapidly grow to form a large mass with cystic spaces, consisting of a jumble of primitive tissues. One type of tissue may outgrow and obscure the others; for example rare tumours occur which appear to consist entirely of thyroid tissue (struma ovarii) and secrete thyroxine, while others resemble choriocarcinoma and secrete hCG.

Endodermal sinus tumour

A very rare highly malignant tumour consisting of yolk-sac endoderm and embryonic mesoblast. It is of interest as it secretes alpha-fetoprotein.

Brenner tumour

This is a small solid benign tumour consisting of fibrous tissue in which isolated epithelial cell nests are scattered, and is thought to arise from epithelial rests which are normally found near the surface of the ovary. Some authorities hold that mucinous cystadenomata arise from the epithelial elements, and ovarian fibromata from the fibrous tissue elements.

Fibroma

A fibroma may be a small nodular growth involving part of the ovary, or the whole organ may be diffusely involved. The diffuse growths are often bilateral, and are smooth oval firm solid tumours with a homogeneous white cut surface. They consist of fusiform connective tissue cells, sometimes with some smooth muscle fibres. They arise from the stroma cells.

Though benign, fibromata are occasionally associated with ascites, and even pleural effusion (Meigs' syndrome).

Granulosa cell tumour

An uncommon tumour that arises most frequently after the menopause, but also both before and during the reproductive period. Its most striking quality is that it secretes oestrogens. After the menopause endometrial proliferation occurs with uterine bleeding. In children precocious uterine bleeding may occur. During the reproductive period there may be irregular bleeding or amenorrhoea.

The tumour is unilateral, solid and seldom large. It consists of granulosa cells resembling those that line the follicle. The cells are small, with deeply staining nuclei, arranged in columns or trabeculae, and often grouped in small rings. About half of the tumours are malignant, though not highly so.

Thecoma

A rarer type of oestrogenic tumour, consisting of cells resembling theca interna cells. Lutein change may occur in both granulosa cell tumours and thecomata.

Androblastoma (arrhenoblastoma)

A very rare tumour that is found in young women, and secretes testosterone in sufficient quantity to produce virilizing effects including amenorrhoea, masculine growth of hair, breast regression and enlargement of the clitoris. It is a small solid tumour that may contain structures resembling imperfect testicular tubules. Usually benign.

Disgerminoma (seminoma)

A rare tumour, most often seen in young adults or children, occasionally in association with testicular feminization (p. 226). It is a solid tumour of moderate size, consisting of groups of large deep-staining cells separated by fibrous septa. The growth is less malignant than seminoma of the testis, which it otherwise resembles. It does not usually secrete hormones.

3. Metastatic carcinoma

Carcinoma may spread to the ovary:

1. From other pelvic sources by lymphatic pathways or peritoneal implant, e.g. from uterine carcinoma.
2. From distant sources, especially from carcinoma of stomach, colon or breast. The Krukenberg tumour is an example, and this arises from a small gastric carcinoma that may be symptomless. Bilateral solid nodular ovarian tumours occur consisting of a cellular stroma in which typical 'signet ring' carcinoma cells are scattered. It is possible that the malignant cells are directly implanted after floating free in the peritoneal cavity, but a lymphatic pathway is also possible.

4. Endometriosis

See p. 298.

Clinical features of ovarian neoplasms

Symptoms

Uncomplicated ovarian cysts are often symptomless, and the first complaint may be of abdominal swelling. Except in bilateral malignant disease some normal ovarian tissue remains, and menstrual disturbance is therefore unusual.*

Pain is infrequent with uncomplicated benign tumours, though large cysts cause abdominal discomfort. Pain occurs with endometriomata and with many complications (described below): torsion, rupture, incarceration, infection, and with malignancy.

Frequency of micturition may occur with a pelvic cyst, or retention of urine if incarceration occurs. Large tumours cause oedema of the legs or vulva.

Signs

An intrapelvic cyst is found on vaginal examination as a rounded mobile painless tumour of fluid consistency, distinct from the uterus, and usually behind it.

Tumours large enough to be felt in the abdomen may lie to one side at first, but come to occupy the midline as they enlarge. A cyst usually rises up out of the pelvis, but it may be possible to push it up far enough to palpate the lower pole abdominally. The tumours are usually smoothly rounded, though some are lobulated. The fluid consistency is obvious except in tense cysts, but in those a fluid thrill may be found. Ovarian tumours are mobile, unless large or complicated. On percussion the tumour is dull, and the flanks are resonant

---

* Granulosa cell tumours, thecoma and androblastoma are rare exceptions to this statement. Uterine bleeding may also occur with endometriosis (p. 298), or with torsion of a cyst, and postmenopausal bleeding may occur with malignant tumours.

(except if there is also ascites) and no souffle is heard on auscultation. The lower pole of a large tumour can be felt vaginally.

The specific endocrine effects of granulosa and theca cell tumours and androblastomata have already been mentioned.

Ultrasound or X-rays may show the outline of a tumour, and in the case of a dermoid cyst teeth may be seen.

Malignant tumours

At operation, 15% of ovarian tumours are found to be malignant, and clinical diagnosis of malignancy is not always possible. Often both ovaries are involved when the case is first seen. These symptoms are suggestive: pain, rapid growth, postmenopausal bleeding. Malignant tumours are often hard and fixed. Ascites is usual, but may also occur with benign fibromata. Secondary deposits in the omentum may be palpable abdominally and deposits in the recto-vaginal pouch may be felt on rectal examination.

Diagnosis

Solid ovarian tumours may be confused with uterine fibromyomata, but the latter often cause menorrhagia, and are hard, multiple and attached to the uterus.

An ovarian cyst may be confused with the pregnant uterus, but in pregnancy amenorrhoea and breast changes occur, the pregnant uterus contracts intermittently, and there is cervical softening. The retroverted gravid uterus may be confused with a cyst, but is continuous with the cervix, which is directed forwards. In difficult cases, especially when pregnancy and a cyst occur together, a hormone test and ultrasonic examination may be useful.

With ascites there is a shifting dullness in the flanks, without a central tumour.

In fat women it may be difficult to exclude an ovarian cyst. With fat there is uniform resistance and dullness, and the umbilicus is deep.

The overfull bladder is certainly diagnosed by passing a catheter.

Inflammatory tubal swellings and pelvic abscess give a characteristic history and signs, and could only be confused with a twisted or infected cyst, though endometriomatous cysts can mimic inflammatory masses.

Screening for ovarian neoplasms. The routine use of high-resolution ultrasound screening will detect any enlargement of the ovary, and laparoscopy can then establish the diagnosis and lead to early treatment.

Complications of ovarian neoplasms

Torsion

Torsion occurs with moderate-sized tumours with long pedicles (e.g. dermoid cyst or fibroma) and is especially common during pregnancy or the puerperium. The cause is obscure. Torsion is often intermittent. The veins in the twisted pedicle are first obstructed, so that the tumour becomes plum coloured and swollen. If the torsion is unrelieved, the arteries then become obliterated, and necrosis and secondary infection of the cyst occurs. Tumours occasionally survive by acquiring a 'parasitic' blood supply from adhesions.

Torsion causes recurrent abdominal pain and vomiting. There may be initial shock, but later there is often slight fever, and sometimes uterine bleeding. The diagnosis depends on the discovery of the rounded tumour.

Rupture

Rupture of a cyst may follow injury or occur spontaneously. The outcome depends on the nature of the cyst. Fluid from a benign cyst is quickly absorbed. Cells from a malignant cyst may be disseminated, or if the cyst is infected, peritonitis will occur. Rupture of a mucinous cyst causes myxoma peritonei (see p. 286). Dermoid cysts rarely rupture, but the contents are highly irritant.

There may be abdominal pain at the time of rupture, and subsequent events depend on the cyst contents. The cyst is not usually palpable after rupture, and with large cysts free fluid may be detected.

Infection

Infection of a cyst may occur by organisms from the bowel after torsion, from the genital tract after delivery, from an infected tube, or after the unwise operation of tapping a cyst. The cyst becomes an abscess, which may point into bowel or bladder, or may burst into the general peritoneal cavity.

Incarceration

A cyst may be held in the pelvis by adhesions, and cause urinary retention as it enlarges.

Complications of pregnancy

Ovarian cysts are often undiagnosed or misdiagnosed when associated with pregnancy. Complications are more common during pregnancy or the puerperium: torsion, rupture, incarceration or infection. The risk of abortion is slightly increased, and a cyst below the presenting part may cause obstructed labour.

Treatment of ovarian neoplasms

Because of the risk of malignancy or of complications, all

ovarian tumours larger than 5 cm in diameter are removed at once. Smaller swellings may be examined by laparascopy. Unless they are follicular or lutein cysts they are removed.

At operation the whole ovary is often removed, but benign tumours can be resected, leaving part of the ovary. The risk of bilateral disease is high, and the opposite ovary is always examined, and in women over 45 should be removed if there is the least abnormality. The second ovary can be split open to examine it, and a biopsy can be taken. For this problem immediate frozen sections are not reliable, and if the later biopsy report shows malignant disease the abdomen should be reopened to remove the second ovary. Tapping of cysts is seldom justifiable to shorten the abdominal incision, as the fear of disseminating malignant cells outweighs the slightly increased risk of hernia with a long incision.

With malignant growths laparatomy should always be performed unless there is obvious remote metastasis. In operable cases the ovaries, tubes and the uterus are removed, and even if this is impossible removal of as much tumour mass as possible will make radiotherapy and chemotherapy more effective. The omentum is a common site for recurrence, and should be removed.

If there are widespread peritoneal deposits radiotherapy is unlikely to help, but it is often used if there is a more localized pelvic mass which cannot be removed. Regression will sometimes occur with chemotherapy, particularly intravenous cisplatin, or oral chlorambucil. In special centres various combinations of drugs are often used. Severe toxic symptoms such as renal damage or depression of bone marrow may occur. Chemotherapy is best given intermittently, e.g. 6 courses of cisplatin infusion over 6 months.

Primary treatment may be followed by a 'second look' laparotomy a few weeks after the primary operation, when localized metastases which have subsequently appeared may be found and either removed or treated with radiation. Such aggressive treatment has improved the prognosis of these cases.

Malignant ascites may sometimes require tapping.

For torsion, rupture or infection, operation is required.

During pregnancy ovarian tumours are removed, though it is justifiable to defer operation during the first 12 weeks for fear of miscarriage. Tumours causing obstructed labour are pushed up above the presenting part if possible, when labour can proceed and the cyst be removed afterwards; but Caesarean section is nearly always required, the cyst being removed after emptying the uterus. Tumours discovered during the puerperium are removed.

TUMOURS OF THE BROAD LIGAMENT

Wolffian cysts

Kobelt's cysts, epoöphoric and paroöphoric cysts are described on p. 219. These are small cysts of little clinical significance.

Fimbrial cysts

These are benign, thin-walled, unilocular cysts that may become 20 cm in diameter. The cysts arise in the broad ligament between the ovary and the tube, and as they enlarge the ovary lies below them, and the greatly elongated tube arches over the cyst. The broad ligament is opened out, and the ureter may be displaced upwards. The cysts contain serous fluid, and are lined by cubical epithelium resembling that of serous ovarian cysts. They sometimes contain papillary processes resembling those in papilliferous ovarian cysts.

The name used here implies that the tumours arise from accessory ovarian tissue that is often found near the fimbria ovarica. Others hold that the cysts arise from the epoöphoron (p. 220).

Large cysts are clinically indistinguishable from ovarian cysts, but small cysts are clearly unilateral and more fixed. The cysts are removed by enucleation, avoiding the ureter.

Fibromyomata

Uterine fibromyomata may grow between the layers of the broad ligament. Fibromyomata may also arise in the broad ligament or round ligament.

Secondary malignant disease

Growths, especially of the cervix, may spread into the broad ligament and may obstruct the ureter.

TUMOURS OF THE UTERINE (FALLOPIAN) TUBE

Benign

Papillomata and fibromyomata are very rare.

Malignant

Carcinoma is very rare. It is usually seen after the menopause and is often bilateral when first discovered. The tubes are distended with growth, either papillary or adenocarcinomatous. Early local and lymphatic spread occurs and the prognosis is very bad. The diagnosis is often missed, but bloodstained watery discharge occurs through the uterus, with pain, and the tubal masses are palpable. When possible hysterectomy and bilateral salpingo-oöphorectomy are performed, and followed by radiotherapy.

ENDOMETRIOSIS

Pathology

The essential feature of endometriosis is the occurrence of endometrial tissue in ectopic situations. An 'endometrioma' may be regarded as a neoplasm, but will only survive under the influence of the ovarian hormones. The ectopic tissue consists of both glands and stroma, in which cyclical menstrual changes occur. The menstrual blood and secretion causes secondary proliferation of adjacent tissue, and the greater part of any tumour is adventitious. Malignant change is very rare indeed. Endometriosis occurs in the following situations:

1. Ovaries. Small dark endometrial 'spots' appear on the surface, and the menstrual secretion distends the endometrial glands and also leaks into the peritoneal cavity, where it is walled off by adhesions. A tumour mass is formed, consisting partly of ovary, partly of adventitious fibrous tissues, and with cystic spaces containing chocolate coloured altered blood. The disease is usually bilateral, and forms masses up to 10 cm in diameter.
2. Uterus. Nodules ('adenomyomata') appear in the wall, resembling fibromyomata, except that they have no definite capsule and show minute spaces containing blood. Microscopically endometrial tissue is found, with proliferation of adjacent muscular and fibrous tissue.
3. Uterine tubes. An uncommon site, except in amputation stumps.
4. Recto-vaginal septum. A hard fixed mass of indefinite outline appears, and may extend backwards partially to surround the rectum. Ulceration of the posterior fornix may occur. The rectal mucosa remains intact for a long time, but ultimately rectal ulceration and bleeding occur. Lateral extension may involve the ureter.

5. Round ligaments, both intra- and extraperitoneal portions.
6. Umbilicus.
7. Lower abdominal scars, especially after hysterotomy.
8. Anywhere on the pelvic peritoneum. Fibrosis related to endometriosis of the bowel may form a ring stricture and cause obstruction. The peritoneal surface of the bladder may be involved.

Aetiological theories

Endometriosis only occurs in tissues adjacent to the Müllerian system. Aetiological theories include:

1. Uterine endometriosis may arise by downgrowth from the endometrium.
2. Endometrial 'spills' may be regurgitated back through the tubes and become implanted. The ovary may be a 'forcing-bed', in which endometriosis may grow, and from which further spills may occur.
3. Endometriosis may result from metaplasia of the coelomic epithelium from which the Müllerian system developed. This may represent an abnormal response to oestrogens.

Symptoms

Endometriosis occurs during the reproductive period, but rarely before 30. Small lesions may be found unexpectedly at operation or at laparoscopy performed for pelvic pain, but larger lesions cause a variety of symptoms:

1. Dysmenorrhoea occurs, and any palpable tumour may become painful at the time of the period. Recto-vaginal lesions cause dyspareunia.
2. Menorrhagia and irregular bleeding occur from associated endometrial hyperplasia or from uterine lesions.
3. Infertility is due to pelvic adhesions or endometrial abnor-

malities. If pregnancy does occur, there is often considerable improvement, at least for a time.
4. Symptoms of intestinal obstruction may occur.

Signs

Physical signs depend on the site of the disease:
1. Ovarian 'chocolate cysts' are tender, fixed, bilateral masses; simulating chronic salpingo-oöphoritis, but without any history of infection, fever or discharge.
2. Uterine lesions cause nodular or uniform uterine enlargement, and may be clinically indistinguishable from fibromyomata or from diffuse hyperplasia.
3. Recto-vaginal lesions are tender, hard, fixed, and simulate rectal carcinoma. In contrast to carcinoma, rectal ulceration is rare and very late.
4. Local lesions (e.g. in scars) may be tender at periods.
5. Endometriosis of bowel may be indistinguishable from carcinoma without histological examination, except that there are often other endometriomatous lesions.

Staging

An international scoring system has been devised. Numerical scores take into account the positions and sizes of the lesions, and the density of adhesions. The purpose is to allow comparison of the results of treatment as assessed by laparoscopy or laparotomy.

Treatment

It was observed that if patients with endometriosis became pregnant their symptoms usually improved, and treatment with progestogens was introduced to produce 'pseudopregnancy', with decidual change and cessation of bleeding in the lesions. Early cases, especially those discovered by laparoscopy, are most suitable. At the time of laparoscopy (or laparotomy) small lesions should be coagulated with a diathermy needle. The patient is then given oral dydrogesterone in increasing doses up to 100 mg daily, continued for 12 months. Treatment with Danazol 200 mg three times daily is now often preferred. This drug binds to progesterone receptors and inhibits formation of oestrogens and adrenal steroids.

A GnRH analogue (Buserelin) which inhibits the output of FSH and LH if it is given daily (p. 329) is under trial.

If symptoms persist after medical treatment laparoscopy should be performed and surgical treatment considered.

If there are chocolate cysts more than 3 cm in diameter these should be excised, and they can often be enucleated without loss of the ovary.

Deposits in the recto-vaginal septum are difficult to treat. If there is no response to hormone treatment surgery is required, but may involve hysterectomy and removal of the ovaries. Operations for intestinal obstruction, or to remove localized deposits from other sites, will occasionally be needed.

18

Functional disorders of menstruation

AMENORRHOEA

Amenorrhoea (absence of menstrual periods) is physiological before puberty, during pregnancy and lactation, and after the menopause. Pathological amenorrhoea is described as false when the flow does not escape because of some obstruction (*cryptomenorrhoea*, p. 222) or true when the endometrial cycle is not occurring.

Aetiology

Patients with amenorrhoea are in two broad groups; those who have never menstruated (primary amenorrhoea), and those in whom the periods have ceased after puberty (secondary amenorrhoea).

Primary amenorrhoea

Primary amenorrhoea occurs in the following conditions, all of which are rare:

1. Pituitary infantilism (Levi-Loraine syndrome). The adult resembles a graceful child. Growth hormone may improve stature, but fertility cannot be achieved.
2. Dystrophia-adiposo-genitalis (Fröhlich syndrome) is characterized by dwarfing, adiposity and genital infantilism.

It is caused by a craniopharyngioma that involves the hypothalamus and pituitary, and requires surgical treatment.
3. Gonadal agenesis (p. 225).
4. Adrenogenital syndrome (p. 226).
5. Untreated cretinism.
6. Congenital failure of uterine development or vaginal atresia.

Except in the last instance the abnormality of development or of general health is the main feature and amenorrhoea is only incidental. It is more common for a doctor to be consulted about delayed puberty in a child with no evident general illness.

Delayed puberty

This may be of serious import. One-third of girls who do not menstruate before the age of 18 may have permanent amenorrhoea. Delayed puberty can arise from any of the disorders listed above, but any disorder of nutrition or general health can affect reproductive function.

The first signs of puberty are proliferation of subareolar mammary tissue and growth of pubic hair. If these are not present by the age of 15 the child should be examined for defective growth or any general disorder. The external genitalia are inspected. If no abnormality is evident it is justifiable to wait 6 months, as many cases prove to be merely 'constitutional', and menstrual periods appear without treatment.

If this does not occur, chromosomal studies are required (p. 223), and rectal and ultrasonic examination to define the size of the ovaries and uterus. Raised serum levels of FSH and LH with low levels of oestrogen suggest ovarian failure. Pituitary activity might be tested by pulsatile administration of GnRH (p. 329). Treatment, if it is possible, is obviously determined by the results of investigation.

Secondary amenorrhoea

This may be caused by:

1. Pituitary disorders:
   a. Pituitary cachexia (Simmonds' disease). Ischaemic necrosis of the pituitary gland may result from thrombosis of pituitary vessels after severe postpartum haemorrhage (p. 163).
   b. Pituitary adenomata secrete prolactin, which blocks the action of gonadotrophins on the ovary. There may be galactorrhoea. X-ray tomography of the pituitary fossa may reveal the tumour, which is often small, although it is occasionally large enough to press on the optic chiasma. Secretion of prolactin can be controlled with bromocriptine 10 mg orally daily, but surgical treatment or radiotherapy is often necessary.
   c. In acromegaly an adenoma of the pituitary may destroy the gonadotrophic cells.
2. Ovarian disorders:
   a. Polycystic ovary syndrome (Stein-Leventhal syndrome) is of unknown cause. After some years of normal menstruation amenorrhoea occurs, sometimes with hirsutes. Both ovaries are enlarged and contain multiple small follicular cysts with hyperplasia of the theca interna, lying in dense stroma. There is no evidence of adrenal disease; the urinary excretion of 17-oxosteroids is normal or only slightly raised. There is a block in the conversion of progesterone to oestrogen, and the intermediate androgenic substance androstenedione appears in excess. In patients with hirsutes plasma testosterone levels are raised. The urinary excretion of oestrogens is normal or low, while that of pregnanetriol (a metabolic product of certain androgens) is raised. The syndrome can be treated with clomiphene (p. 325) or GnRH.

b. Androblastoma is a very rare cause of amenorrhoea.
c. Irradiation or excision of the ovaries causes amenorrhoea, but infection or new growths seldom do so, because such disorders are unlikely to destroy all ovarian tissue. If amenorrhoea occurs with malignant disease or tuberculosis general ill-health is usually the cause rather than destruction of the ovary.

3. Uterine disease:
The endometrium atrophies after irradiation.
4. Other endocrine disorders:
    a. Severe hypo- or hyperthyroidism.
    b. Severe diabetes.
    c. Addison's disease.
    d. Adrenocortical tumour or hyperplasia. Apart from cases of the adrenogenital syndrome (see p. 226) an excess of androgens may be produced in adult life by tumours or hyperplasia of the suprarenal cortex. With the amenorrhoea there is hirsutes and enlargement of the clitoris. There will be an excess of oxosteroids in the urine. The treatment is surgical.

    In Cushing's syndrome there is also cortical hyperplasia or tumour, but in this syndrome there is chiefly an excess of glucocorticoids. The patients are obese, often with cutaneous striae, hirsutes, hypertension, osteoporosis and diabetes. Surgical treatment may be possible.
5. Nervous disorders (stress or hypothalamic amenorrhoea). This is the commonest type of secondary amenorrhoea, and may be the result of emotional disturbance (e.g. the stress of a new environment). It also occurs with many longstanding psychiatric disorders, especially depression or anxiety states. In cases of anorexia nervosa amenorrhoea often occurs.
6. Disorders of general health and nutrition. Any chronic or severe illness may cause amenorrhoea.

7. Oral contraception. A delayed first period is common after stopping oral contraception. More prolonged amenorrhoea sometimes occurs. This is unrelated to the type of pill or length of use, and usually recovers spontaneously. There is often a history of irregular periods before starting oral contraception. The possibility of pregnancy must not be forgotten.

Investigation of secondary amenorrhoea. During the reproductive period pregnancy is the commonest cause of amenorrhoea; otherwise a local pelvic cause is rare. In diagnosis general health is first considered, including psychological and environmental factors.

Hormone assays are now available in many laboratories. Radioimmunoasaay of prolactin and FSH in serum should be performed. The prolactin concentration should be less than 580 mIU/L, but a higher level should not be accepted as correct without repetition, because stress can raise the level. Levels above 1000 mIU/L call for treatment.

The history or examination may suggest the need for other hormonal assays, and Table 18.1 shows some of the results which can be obtained.

Withdrawal bleeding after administration of a progestogen such as norethisterone 15 mg daily by mouth for 5 days will prove that the endometrium is responsive.

Treatment of secondary amenorrhoea. Amenorrhoea may be a symptom of one of the disorders already described which requires treatment on its own account, but if this is not the case it is pointless to give treatment for the amenorrhoea unless the patient wishes for pregnancy either immediately or in the future. Many cases of secondary amenorrhoea are temporary and recover spontaneously, but if amenorrhoea persists for longer than a year there is a risk of it becoming permanent. The elimination of stress and emotional factors. or correction of an inadequate diet, may be all that is required.

Table 18.1 Some typical results of investigations in cases of amenorrhoea or of failure of ovulation

	Menses	Endometrium	Pituitary fossa	Ovarian ultrasound	Plasma gonadotrophins	Plasma oestrogens	
Pituitary failure	Absent	Atrophic	Normal	Normal	Low	Low	
Ovarian dysfunction	Absent	Atrophic	Normal	Normal	High	Low	
Adrenal hyperplasia or tumour	Absent	Normal	Normal	Normal	Normal	Normal	Oxosteroids high in urine
Polycystic ovary (Stein-Leventhal) syndrome	Absent	Hyperplasia	Normal	Small cysts	LH raised FSH normal or raised	Normal	Pregnanetriol raised in urine. If hirsute, testosterone raised in plasma.
Pituitary prolactinoma	Absent	Atrophic	Enlarged	Normal	FSH normal low LH Normal	Low	Prolactin raised in plasma
Cyclic anovular bleeding	Apparently normal	Non-secretory	Normal	Normal	or low	Normal	
Irregular anovular bleeding	Irregular	Hyperplastic	Normal	Normal or small cysts	Normal	High and erratic	

If the hormone levels and the ovaries are normal, and withdrawal bleeding takes place after giving a progestogen, then induction of ovulation with clomiphene (p. 325), gonadotrophins or GnRH (p. 326) may be considered.

ANOVULAR MENSTRUATION

Sometimes in a menstrual cycle ovulation does not occur, and the endometrium does not undergo secretory change. Such cycles may be short, 21 to 24 days in length, and are characteristically painless. The loss is not usually abnormal, but in a few cases endometrial ripening is erratic, and the period is prolonged (see below).

Anovular cycles may occur at the menarche until regular ovulation is established, and with increasing frequency after the age of 40. Such cycles are found in a third of women complaining of infertility.

The diagnosis is confirmed by finding a flat basal temperature chart (p. 322), with low plasma progesterone levels, and non-secretory endometrium in a premenstrual biopsy. Treatment is only necessary if pregnancy is desired, when ovulation can be induced by the methods described on p. 325.

DYSFUNCTIONAL UTERINE BLEEDING

This term has been contrived to include cases of abnormal uterine bleeding other than those caused by complications of pregnancy, gross lesions of the uterus such as fibromyomata, tubo-ovarian lesions such as salpingitis or endometriosis, or intrauterine contraceptive devices. Although dysfunctional bleeding is common its explanation is often obscure. The cases can be divided into those with non-ovulatory cycles and those with ovulatory cycles.

Non-ovulatory bleeding

(1) A well-recognized syndrome is that of *cystic glandular*

hyperplasia of the endometrium (formerly known as metropathia haemorrhagica). It is believed that the normal inhibitory feedback of the hypothalamo-pituitary unit by ovarian oestrogens fails, and the output of oestrogen from the ovarian follicles rises erratically to high levels. There are often follicular cysts in the ovaries.

As ovulation does not occur no progesterone is produced by the ovary and there are no secretory changes in the endometrium. The continued unopposed action of oestrogens causes abnormal hyperplasia of the endometrium, which becomes thickened and polypoid. It often contains cystic glands, giving a 'Swiss cheese' appearance, with small areas of necrosis. The myometrium is also hypertrophied, so that the uterus is slightly enlarged.

There is commonly an initial phase of 6–8 weeks' amenorrhoea, followed by irregular bleeding.

(2) Many women with regular anovulatory cycles (see above) have no excessive bleeding, but in a few cases the endometrium is shed irregularly and incompletely with prolonged or excessive loss.

Ovulatory bleeding

Abnormal bleeding sometimes occurs although ovulation has taken place and the endometrium shows some secretory changes. This may be because luteal function is inadequate and hormone levels are lower than normal in the late cycle, and endometrial ripening is deficient.

Alternatively the corpus luteum may persist longer than normal, so that the secretory endometrium is shed irregularly, with prolonged or heavy loss.

Prostaglandins

The theories outlined above relate to levels of gonadotrophic and ovarian hormones. Recently prostaglandin synthesis in the endometrium has also been implicated. In normal cycles the PG content of endometrium is highest at the time of menstruation. The part played by PGs in dysfunctional bleeding is still uncertain.

$PGF_{2\alpha}$ causes vasoconstriction and myometrial contraction, PGE_2 is a vasodilator, and prostacyclin causes myometrial relaxation and is a vasodilator. It is stated that in menorrhagia there is a decrease in $PGF_{2\alpha}$ relative to PGE_2, and inhibitors of prostaglandin synthetase have been used in treatment, with some, but not uniform, success.

Clinical features and management

Many cases resolve spontaneously after a few cycles, and any claim that improvement is the result of treatment must be considered critically. It is convenient to subdivide the cases according to the ages of the patients.

Menorrhagia of puberty

This is relatively rare. In initial cycles ovulation may not occur, and with the unbalanced action of oestrogens early periods may be profuse. Excessive bleeding usually ceases spontaneously after a few cycles, and undue attention to it gives a child an undesirable impression of abnormality. If, however, abnormal bleeding continues clomiphene citrate 50 mg may be given for 5 days, starting on the first day of bleeding. This causes an increased output of gonadotrophins.

Precocious puberty

Although this is not part of dysfunctional bleeding, it is convenient to mention it here. In most cases ovarian and uterine structure and function are normal, and such 'constitutional' cases do not require treatment. Rarely precocious bleeding may be caused by a granulosa cell tumour of the ovary, or by encephalitis or a tumour affecting the hypothalamus.

Dysfunctional bleeding during the reproductive period

All the varieties of dysfunctional bleeding described above may occur. Sometimes patients give dramatic accounts of heavy loss which direct observation in hospital does not confirm; if the haemoglobin level can be maintained with iron little else may be necessary. With severe bleeding diagnostic curetting is performed, chiefly to exclude other lesions, and it is wise before complicated endocrine therapy. Curetting is primarily diagnostic, and if an endocrine imbalance persists the bleeding will recur. Rest in bed may temporarily control excessive bleeding. Oxytocin or ergometrine is of little use.

Endocrine treatment. Irregular or excessive bleeding with anovular cycles may be treated with progestogens, with the aim of inducing or increasing luteal changes. Norethisterone 15 mg orally is given from the 10th to the 25th day; if the bleeding is irregular the course has to be started at random. After stopping the progestogen withdrawal bleeding occurs, but hopefully in slighter amount. The treatment may have to continue for several cycles.

Alternatively an oral contraceptive containing a high dose of progestogen is given from the 5th to the 21st day, e.g. Gynovlar or Microgynon.

For the patient who also complains of infertility induction of ovulation (p. 325) is advised.

Another method of treatment is to give a GnRH analogue continuously (not intermittently). This will inhibit the output of gonadotrophins and therefore of ovarian hormones (p. 329).

Treatment by inhibition of prostaglandin synthesis. Drugs such as mefenamic acid (Ponstan) 500 mg three times daily before and during menstruation are effective in some cases, but unpredictably.

Surgical treatment. In persistent cases hysterectomy may be performed, with conservation of the ovaries in premenopausal women. As an alternative the endometrium can be destroyed with a laser beam directed through a fibreoptic system which is passed through a hysteroscope.

Premenopausal cases

After ovulation and progesterone production cease at the menopause, oestrogen is still produced for a time, and its unopposed action may cause endometrial hyperplasia with excessive or irregular bleeding. This is a condition of limited duration, but its chief importance is in diagnosis. Curetting is essential to exclude malignant disease. In some cases bleeding does not recur after curetting, but if it does hysterectomy is performed.

DYSMENORRHOEA

Dysmenorrhoea, or painful menstruation, is difficult to define precisely as many healthy women have some menstrual discomfort. Probably 3% of women have sufficient pain to seek some sort of treatment, and in about half of these the pain is enough to interrupt work. Dysmenorrhoea may be primary or secondary.

Secondary dysmenorrhoea

This is caused by such conditions as fibromyomata, endometriosis or salpingo-oöphoritis, and occurs after some years of painless periods. It may be (a) congestive, due to inflammatory disease or endometriosis or (b) less commonly spasmodic, due to uterine contractions while expelling a fibromyomatous polyp or blood clot. Laparoscopy may reveal early lesions of endometriosis that are not palpable on ordinary examination.

Primary dysmenorrhoea

This is far more common than secondary dysmenorrhoea. Pain is only felt in ovulatory cycles, and the first few cycles after the menarche may be painless. The pain coincides with spasmodic uterine contractions, and is probably ischaemic as the uterus contracts strongly enough to shut off its own circulation temporarily. It usually ceases after bearing a child, and is sometimes relieved by dilating the cervix. Similar pain is produced by stimulation of the region of the internal os, when uterine contractions are induced.

Aetiological theories:
1. Although it has been stated that dysmenorrhoeic uteri are hypoplastic, this is untrue.
2. Endocrine abnormalities have not been found; fertility is normal.
3. Prostaglandins from disintegrating endometrium may cause uterine spasm. In cases of dysmenorrhoea the concentration of $PGF_{2\alpha}$ in menstrual fluid is increased.
4. Psychological factors may accentate symptoms, especially in a child who is led to expect menstrual disability.

Symptoms. There is intermittent pain, which accompanies the flow, and rarely lasts more than a few hours. The pain is felt in the back and lower abdomen, sometimes radiating down the thighs.

Treatment. The incidence of dysmenorrhoea in girls has been reduced by sensible education, and by avoiding unnecessary restriction of activity during a period.

Pain-relieving drugs are given in full doses, but habit-forming drugs are avoided. Paracetamol tablets (up to 1 g three times daily) are popular. This drug is combined with dextropropoxyphene in Distalgesic tablets. Dihydrocodeine tablets (30 mg 4-hourly) are also used. Antispasmodics are usually ineffective. Whatever pain-relieving drugs are used should be given in full doses. To restore confidence it is essential to break the sequence of painful periods.

Relief may be obtained with drugs which block prostaglandin production, such as mefenamic acid (Ponstan) 500 mg three times daily. These drugs must be used carefully, as they will adversely affect some other medical disorders, including asthma.

An alternative treatment is to inhibit ovulation. This is achieved with a high-progestogen low-oestrogen combined pill (see p. 337). Another progestogen, dydrogesterone (Duphaston), will relieve pain without inhibiting ovulation; 10 mg daily is given orally from the 5th to the 25th day of the cycle.

Dilatation of the cervix under anaesthesia cures about a quarter of the cases but this treatment carries the risk of damaging the cervix, and causing miscarriage in a subsequent pregnancy. In exceptional and severe cases 'presacral' neurectomy is performed. Through a lower abdominal incision the hypogastric plexus is divided where it lies in the retroperitoneal tissue in front of the last lumbar vertebra.

Intermenstrual pain

Pain at mid-cycle (for which the fatuous term 'Mittelschmerz' is often used) is sometimes attributed to ovulation. It is true that in rare cases free haemorrhage may occur from a follicle, but this is not repeated in each cycle. If an accurate calendar is kept a diagnosis of repeated ovulatory pain will often be abandoned.

Premenstrual tension (see p. 12)

Symptoms may be relieved by giving diuretics such as chlorothiazide in the premenstrual week. Strong claims have been made for the effectiveness of oral progestogens, such as norethisterone 20 mg daily from the 15th to the 25th day of the cycle, but tranquillizers, such as meprobamate 200 mg thrice daily, with sympathy and emotional support, appear to be equally effective.

19

Menopausal symptoms

The physiological events at the menopause have been mentioned on p. 14. Many women have symptoms at this time for which they may seek advice.

Menopausal flushes

About half of all menopausal women notice hot flushes. There is a sudden sensation of heat, most commonly over the face, neck, chest and arms, associated with sweating, and lasting for some minutes. It can be shown that there is peripheral vasodilatation, and sometimes a change in heart rate. A few flushes may be accepted by the woman as a temporary inconvenience, but sometimes the flushes are very frequent and persistent.

Chiefly because they can be relieved by oestrogens the flushes have been attributed to the menopausal fall in ovarian hormones. Flushes may occur after oöphorectomy. However, flushes do not occur before puberty nor in conditions such as ovarian agenesis in which oestrogen levels are low, except after administration and subsequent withdrawal of oestrogens.

Flushes cannot be attributed to the high levels of gonadotrophins at the menopause, as high levels often persist after the flushes have ceased, and flushes are not produced by gonadotrophin therapy or administration of GnRH.

It seems evident that the cause must be sought in readjustment of the local or central mechanism for vasomotor control, and the relationship between oestrogens and catecholamines is now being investigated.

Flushes are treated with oestrogens. Premarin, an oestrogen of equine origin, may be given orally (1.25 mg daily) but probably has no advantage over ethinyl oestradiol (10 micrograms daily). Another preparation in use is piperazine oestrone sulphate (Harmogen), 3 mg daily for 21 out of each 28 days. The dosage of all these preparations is adjusted according to the effect on the flushes, and usually discontinued after about 6 months.

Long-term treatment at the menopause

Apart from the relatively short-term treatment of flushes, some doctors regard the menopause as an endocrine deficiency disease for which long-term treatment is required.

Coronary thrombosis is much less common in women than in men before the age of 50, after which the incidence becomes more equal, and it is suggested that oestrogens protect women from arterial disease. After the menopause osteoporosis is more common and progresses more rapidly in women than in men. Bone loss can be reduced by treatment with oestrogen, and if this is continued for many years the incidence of vertebral, femoral and other fractures may be reduced.

Emotional depression may also occur at menopausal age, although it is just as likely to be the result of changing circumstances in life as of hormonal alteration. Because of these various clinical facts some doctors prescribe oestrogens as hormonal replacement therapy for an indefinite time after the menopause.

The oestrogens are given daily, but if they are taken continuously they may cause irregular endometrial bleeding, with a risk of endometrial carcinoma and of diagnostic confusion. A progestogen is therefore also prescribed, such as norethisterone 5 mg daily for the first 14 days of each month, and endometrial bleeding follows regularly. The progestogen need not be given to any woman who has had a hysterectomy.

As an alternative to daily medication a subcutaneous implant of oestradiol-17β, 50 mg, is sometimes used. It is effective for 4 to 6 months before replacement is needed.

However, the majority of women do not want perpetual treatment, and most doctors still prefer to use oestrogens to treat any menopausal symptoms, and then gradually reduce and discontinue them.

Other menopausal conditions

In a few women atrophic changes occur in the vulval epithelium (*atrophic vulvitis*, p. 243). Ascending infection may occur when the vaginal acidity falls after the menopause, causing *atrophic vaginitis* (p. 247) or *atrophic endometritis* (p. 251). These conditions will respond to treatment with oestrogens.

Dysfunctional uterine bleeding may occur near the time of the menopause, but from unbalanced action rather than lack of oestrogens.

20

Dyspareunia

Dyspareunia means painful coitus. If pain persists after any initial hymeneal laceration has healed it is termed *primary dyspareunia*. This may be due to a resistant hymen, a narrow introitus, or very rarely to some congenital abnormality. More often there is no anatomical abnormality, but the difficulty is caused by contraction of the perineal muscles (*vaginismus*), due to psychological eversion, and the patient has never allowed penetration. In such cases emotional problems will need discussion. A course of relaxation exercises, as described by Kegel, will usually cure vaginismus.

With inadequate or unskilful sexual stimulation vaginal and vestibular secretion is lacking, and soreness may ensue. Advice to the partner and the use of a simple lubricant may help. Only if there is real organic narrowing should a plastic operation (p. 222) be recommended. Alternately the patient may use a set of graduated vaginal dilators. In the majority of cases emotional difficulties are the basic problem. Advice about the choice of a contraceptive method may be needed.

If dyspareunia appears after previous painless intercourse it is termed *secondary*. Treatment is directed to the cause, which is usually a local lesion, although it may have a psychological basis. Pain at the introitus may be due to: caruncle, acute vulvitis, Bartholinitis, a tender perineal scar, atrophic vulvitis. Deep tenderness may be caused by salpingitis or endometriosis.

21

Infertility

Because of the complexity of human reproductive physiology the causes of infertility are numerous. If a couple have never achieved pregnancy at any time the infertility is described as *primary*; if infertility follows a pregnancy, whatever the outcome, it is called *secondary*. Conception occurs after varying intervals because of many factors, such as age, frequency of intercourse, regularity of ovulation, freedom from ill health and stress, but more than 80% of couples will achieve pregnancy during one year of trying.

Male factors

In about 15% of sterile marriages the male is wholly at fault, and he is partly at fault in a large number. Unlike the female, who is born with her total complement of eggs, the male produces sperm more or less continuously, each 'wave' of spermatozoa taking 72 days to mature. Spermatogenesis can be depressed by many factors, including excessive smoking or alcohol consumption, and overwork. If the scrotal temperature is raised by a varicocele or the wearing of thick underpants low sperm counts (oligospermia) may occur. Failure of descent of the testes leads to azoospermia. If the testes are small or absent chromosomal investigations must be made.

Seminal examination is important. The specimen is

obtained by masturbation into a sterile glass or plastic vessel (not rubber). It should be analysed immediately. A normal specimen measures 2 ml or more, and contains more than 20 000 000 sperms per ml, of which more than 75% are motile. The direction of movement is important; the majority of sperm should show progressive forward movement as opposed to random movements. Less than 25% should be abnormally formed. Absent or low motility or numerous abnormal forms (usually immature spermatids) are more serious findings than a low count.

Seminal fluid contains both sperms and plasma. Biochemical investigation of the plasma gives an index of the function of the male accessory glands. Fructose, from the seminal vesicle, provides for the energy requirements of the spermatozoa. Phosphate, from the prostate, and glyceryl phosphoryl choline, from the epididymis, can also be measured. If all these are normal the vas deferens must be patent and accessory gland function is normal.

The seminal fluid analysis should be repeated at least once and after a 14 day interval to obtain reliable results.

In addition a sperm penetration test (p. 323) or a postcoital examination of the cervical mucus for the presence of sperms may be made (p. 323).

Impotence, premature ejaculation and infrequent intercourse are obvious cause of infertility.

Female factors

There are many causes of female infertility.

Ovulation

Regular ovulation is clearly essential for fertility. Regular menses suggest regular ovulation, but anovular cycles are found in one third of women who complain of infertility

(p. 308). In any severe illness or nutritional disturbance, or in specific endocrine disorders, ovulation and menstruation may cease.

Local pelvic lesions may interfere with the passage of the egg into or along the uterine tube, or with fertilization by the sperm; for example pelvic inflammatory lesions, endometriosis, or other gross ovarian disease.

Ovulation occurs at about the 14th day of the normal cycle, and conception is most likely with intercourse at or shortly before this time.

Confirmation of ovulation is obtained by the following investigations:

1. The basal body temperature, taken orally on waking (and best plotted on a chart) by the patient, shows a rise of more than 0.5°C at ovulation which is sustained during the luteal phase.
2. An endometrial biopsy, taken without anaesthesia with a fine suction curette during the second half of the cycle, will show luteal changes, but this is now seldom done as the growth and rupture of the follicle can be followed with repeated ultrasound observations.
3. A plasma progesterone concentration greater than 15 mmol/l on the 21st day of the cycle indicates normal corpus luteum function.

Transit of sperms and egg

Vaginal and cervical function. Spermatozoa soon die in the acid vaginal secretion. The spermatozoa are initially protected by coagulation of seminal fluid in the vagina, because of fibrinogen in the seminal plasma. They then enter the alkaline cervical mucus which is present at the time of ovulation. Incomplete coitus is therefore less likely to effect fertilization, and dyspareunia or vaginal obstruction may cause sterility. The female can conceive in the absence of orgasm, but sexual stimuli may increase fertility by increasing alkaline cervical secretion. Cervical mucus is a complex hydrogel which is opaque, viscid and small in amount during the first ten days of the cycle. Under the influence of oestrogens produced by the ovarian follicle in the days leading up to ovulation the mucus becomes copious, clear and less viscid, so that it can be drawn out into a fine thread. It shows fern-like patterns of salt crystals when it is dried on a microscope slide. Sperms can more easily penetrate ovulatory mucus. After ovulation the mucus becomes viscid again and ferning is not seen. After high cervical amputation, infertility may occur, not only because of increased risk of abortion, but because of altered cervical secretion.

It is important to establish the compatibility of sperm and cervical mucus. In the Sims-Huhner *post-coital test* mucus from the cervical canal is examined within a few hours of intercourse. The test is only valid with ovulatory mucus. The number of motile and actively progressing sperm are counted: more than 10 should be found in a high-power field. A positive result proves that male function is satisfactory and also excludes a cervical factor in infertility. If no sperms or only dead sperms are found further investigation is needed. Because there is little correlation between the results of postcoital tests and the occurrence of pregnancy they are now often replaced by *sperm penetration tests*, in which a sample of fresh semen is placed in a small tube containing the cervical mucus, and the penetration by the sperm is observed. Death of the sperm on entering the mucus may be due to antibodies. This possibility can be investigated further by a crossed sperm penetration test, in which the husband's sperm is tested with normal donor cervical mucus, and the wife's cervical mucus with normal donor sperm. Sperm antibodies can also be investigated by analysis of blood serum.

Tubal function. The egg is normally fertilized in the uterine tube; obviously tubal blockage prevents conception. Blockage is usually due to salpingitis, including tuberculous salpingitis, which may be clinically latent. Salpingitis may not only block the tubes but also damage the ciliated epithelium. Adhesions from this or other pelvic inflammatory disease may kink the tubes, or cover the fimbrial ends of the tubes or the surfaces of the ovaries.

Tubal patency is best tested by laparoscopy (p. 368). A solution of methylene blue is injected from a cannula in the cervical canal, and filling of the tubes and spill of the dye from the abdominal ostia is directly observed. Laparoscopy also allows inspection of the peritoneal surfaces and the ovaries. An additional procedure is to examine the uterine cavity and internal tubal openings by hysteroscopy (p. 369).

A procedure which is now less often used is hysterosalpingography. In this 10 to 20 ml of water-soluble radio-opaque dye is injected through a cervical cannula and the outline of the uterine cavity and tubes can be seen on the X-ray screen.

Tests for tubal patency should not be done in the presence of active pelvic infection.

Embedding and maintenance of the embryo

Ill-health, malnutrition and specific endocrine disorders will disturb the menstrual rhythm. Not only may ovulation cease, but the premenstrual preparation for the reception of the ovum may be inadequate. Commonly there is amenorrhoea or altered rhythm, but even with normal rhythm it is possible that in some cases insufficient progesterone is produced to maintain the early decidua.

Failure of embedding or early abortion may be due to local uterine disease, such as congenital hypoplasia, polypi, or fibromyomata.

Investigation and treatment of the infertile couple

In young people it is sensible to start investigation after 18 months of infertility, but with older patients earlier investigation is justifiable. After taking a detailed history and making a clinical examination of both partners the following routine tests are made:

1. Confirmation of ovulation (p. 322).
2. Seminal fluid analysis (at least two tests) (p. 321).
3. Sperm penetration test or post-coital test (p. 323).
4. Tests for tubal patency (p. 368).

In most cases no abnormality is found, and with reassurance pregnancy will soon follow. If an abnormality is discovered then further treatment may be required.

1. *Failure to ovulate.* Ovulation may be induced with clomiphene, gonadotrophins and, recently, gonadotrophin releasing hormone.

Clomiphene citrate inhibits the negative feedback of ovarian hormones on the hypothalamus, and thus causes an increased output of gonadotrophins. A daily dose of 50 mg is taken orally during the first 5 days of the menstrual cycle, and ovulation may occur about 10 days after the completion of treatment. If there is no response the dose is gradually increased, up to 200 mg daily. The treatment must be monitored (see below).

Gonadotrophins. As it is not possible to obtain adequate supplies of extracts of human pituitary glands, an extract of human menopausal urine (hMG) is used. This contains FSH and LH. Intramuscular injections of hMG are given over 7 to 10 days to produce follicular ripening, and are followed by an injection of 5000 units of human chorionic gonadotrophin. This acts like LH and induces ovulation in the ripe follicle. The usual starting dose of hMG is 375 units daily. If there is no response the dose is progressively increased up to 1500 units daily. The patient's response must be carefully monitored (see below), otherwise overstimulation will result in multiple ovulation and multiple pregnancies, or the formation of large haemorrhagic ovarian follicles, with severe abdominal pain.

Gonadotrophin releasing hormone (GnRH). This has largely replaced gonadotrophins for induction of ovulation. A small pump is strapped to the patient's arm to administer a pulse of 20 micrograms of GnRH subcutaneously every 90 minutes. Treatment is continued for 10 days until a ripe follicle is produced. An injection of chorionic gonadotrophin is then given, to induce ovulation.

Monitoring of induced ovulation. Ultrasonic monitoring of the enlargement of the ovarian follicle is essential to prevent overstimulation and to judge when to give hCG. Provided that the results can be obtained in less than 24 hours, assays of blood levels of oestradiol and LH are also useful.

Amenorrhoea and failure of ovulation caused by hyperprolactinaemia is treated with bromocriptine (p. 304).

2. *Tubal damage* accounts for about 15% of cases of infertility. In cases caused by salpingitis the degree of damage to the ciliated epithelium and the muscular wall of the tube determines the prognosis. Simple peritubal adhesions are freed by operation (salpingolysis). Adherent fimbriae can often be separated easily. It is not difficult to make a new opening into the tube (salpingostomy), but the pregnancy rate is less than 10% because of previous damage to the ciliated epithelium. More difficult operations include excision of a stricture and end-to-end anastomosis, or excision of the interstitial part of the tube and reimplantation of the uterine end. Fine instruments and an operating microscope are required.

Reversal of sterilization is sometimes requested. If the tube has only been occluded with a clip there is fair hope of success.

Even if pregnancy follows tubal surgery there is a risk that this will be ectopic.

Extracorporeal fertilization (*in vitro fertilization*) of an oöcyte is possible for patients with blocked tubes. Maturation of the ovarian follicle is followed with serial ultrasonic measurements, and when it is ripe the oöcyte is aspirated from it with a needle passed through the abdominal wall under ultrasound control. After a few hours incubation the oöcyte is exposed to spermatozoa while under observation with a microscope. The fertilized ovum is cultured for 48 hours and then inserted into the uterus through the cervix. To increase the success rate, multiple ovulation may be induced with clomiphene or gonadotrophins. However, not more than three of the embryos should be implanted because of the risk of multiple pregnancy.

3. *Hostile cervical mucus.* Ethinyl oestradiol 10 micrograms orally daily for 3 days before ovulation may improve the consistency of the mucus.

There is at present no certain method of treating antibody reaction to the sperm.

4. *Other gynaecological abnormalities* such as fibromyomata, endometriosis or cervical incompetence may require treatment. Uncomplicated retroversion or cervical erosion are not causes of infertility.

5. *Coital problems.* Advice on normal coital behaviour is sometimes necessary, and also about the timing of intercourse in relation to ovulation.

6. *Oligospermia.* Simple measures such as taking cold baths and wearing loose underwear may be effective. Improvement may follow operative cure of a varicocele.

Treatment with androgens (Mesterolone 25 mg orally four times daily) is often given. It must be continued for at least 6 months, because of the long cycle of spermatogenesis. However, the treatment of oligospermia is disappointing, less than a third of the couples achieving a pregnancy. Artificial insemination with husband's semen (AIH) can be performed by injection of fresh semen into the cervical canal with a small syringe and cannula; this might ensure that more sperm reach the uterine cavity, but it is of doubtful value.

7. *Azoospermia*. If this is caused by a chromosomal abnormality no treatment is possible. Insemination with donor semen (AID) is often successful in achieving pregnancy. Adequate counselling is essential, and legal points may arise. Adoption or fostering may be an alternative solution.

A few cases result from blockage of the vas or epididymal tubules and surgical treatment is possible, but with small hope of success.

22

Endocrine preparations

Endocrine treatment has an important place in gynaecology. It is not intended that the student should memorize the chemical formulae given in this chapter; their purpose is only to aid understanding.

Hypothalamic gonadotrophin-releasing hormone (GnRH)

This is a decapeptide which releases both FSH and LH and is effective in inducing ovulation if it is given in intermittent pulses. For this purpose it is administered subcutaneously by means of a small pump which is attached to the patient's arm (p. 326).

If it is given continuously GnRH *inhibits* the secretion of FSH and LH by pituitary cells, and therefore the levels of ovarian hormones fall and amenorrhoea occurs.

Synthetic analogues of GnRH are now available in which one or more of the amino acids in natural GnRH have been changed. The analogues bind more strongly to pituitary receptors and have a longer half-life than natural GnRH. They can be given by subcutaneous injection or intranasally, e.g. Buserelin 200 micrograms s.c. or 1000 micrograms i.u. daily. Because their action is more prolonged and therefore more continuous than that of the natural hormone they are less suitable for induction of ovulation, but their powerful effect in suppressing oestrogen secretion makes them suitable for treatment of endometriosis (p. 298), dysfunctional endometrial bleeding (p. 308) or fibromyomata (p. 264). Although synthetic GnRH analogues inhibit ovulation and could therefore be used for contraception they are not recommended for this purpose as they cause amenorrhoea or irregular periods.

Pituitary gonadotrophic hormones (FSH and LH)

These are glycoproteins which can be measured by radioimmunoassay in units based on international standard preparations. Both hormones can be extracted from human pituitary glands, but obviously the supply from this source is limited, and gonadotrophins are usually obtained from extracts of human menopausal urine. Such preparations (hMG) contain both FSH and LH, and can be used to induce ovulation (p. 325).

Chorionic gonadotrophin (hCG)

This is extracted from pregnancy urine or placentae. Although it differs from LH the two substances have similar biological activity and hCG will cause ovulation from a ripe follicle.

Ovarian steroids

Oestrogens, progesterone and androgens are all found in varying amounts in the adrenal cortex, testis, ovary and placenta. There is a common biochemical pathway by which they are formed:

$$\text{Cholesterol} \to \text{progesterone} \begin{array}{l} \to \text{androgens} \to \text{oestrogens} \\ \to \text{corticosteroids} \end{array}$$

The various ovarian steroids share a basic chemical structure, in which each carbon atom is given a conventional number, and some of these are indicated below.

Oestrogens

Oestradiol 17β is secreted by the ovarian follicle, and during pregnancy by the placenta. It is partly metabolized to *oestrone* and *oestriol* and excreted in the urine. The natural hormones are relatively inactive when given by mouth. Oestrogens in plasma may be free or bound to protein. They are measured in plasma by radioimmunoassay, and chemical assay is possible for urinary samples which contain large amounts of oestrogens.

Synthetic modifications which are active by mouth include *17 β ethinyl oestradiol* and *mestranol*. Both can be used for oral contraception. Other synthetic oestrogens such as *diethyl stilboestrol* are also active by mouth, but their chemical structure is unrelated to that of the natural hormones.

Premarin is a proprietary preparation of conjugated oestrogens derived from the serum of pregnant mares.

Oestrogens are absorbed through the vaginal epithelium,

and are sometimes administered as vaginal pessaries or cream. For patients who have had the uterus and ovaries removed oestradiol can be implanted subcutaneously to give a slow release over several weeks.

Oestrogens can be used:

1. To inhibit ovulation. Oral contraceptive pills contain oestrogens (p. 337), and these pills can also be used to treat dysmenorrhoea (p. 312).
2. For menopausal flushes (p. 316).
3. To induce maturation of the epithelium of the lower genital tract in vulvo-vaginitis of children, primary atrophy of the vulva, atrophic vaginitis and endometritis.
4. To modify cervical mucus.

Progestogens

Progesterone is inactive when given orally, but many synthetic compounds have been introduced which are active by mouth. Although all of these have some progestogenic activity, their actions differ from those of progesterone and may include some oestrogenic and androgenic effects.

PROGESTERONE

A few selected examples of progestogens will be mentioned:
Derivatives of nortestosterone. If the methyl group at C19 in testosterone is replaced by an H atom we have nortestosterone, and by adding an ethinyl group at C17 *norethisterone* is produced. This is active by mouth, has some oestrogenic action, inhibits ovulation, and is effective in controlling

endometrial bleeding. It does not produce an ordinary secretory endometrium, but an unusual type of proliferation.

Derivatives of progesterone. By attaching an ethinyl group at C17, with various other alterations in the side chains, *levonorgestrel, desogestrel, gestadine, norgestimate* and *gestrinone* are produced, all of which are active by mouth.

Another modification of progesterone is to attach a hexanoate group at C17, to give *17α hydroxyprogesterone hexanoate* (Primolut D) which is slowly absorbed after intramuscular injection. It may be used in cases of endometrial cancer.

Dydrogesterone (Duphaston) is a stereoisomer of progesterone. It has no oestrogenic activity, and is claimed not to inhibit ovulation. It has been used for the treatment of dysmenorrhoea and endometriosis.

In summary, the various progestogens have been used in oral contraceptives, and for treatment of dysmenorrhoea, premenstrual tension, dysfunctional bleeding, endometriosis and endometrial cancer.

23

Contraception, sterilization and termination of pregnancy

In the United Kingdom more than five million women seek family planning advice in each year, and such advice is an important part of gynaecological practice. It is not only for the benefit of the individual woman, but is of world-wide importance. If the present rate of reproduction continues the world population could double in the next century. Infanticide is unacceptable; repeated abortion is not without danger to life and health; proper contraceptive advice is safer for the woman and cheaper for the nation.

The large number of abortions in Britain prove that many women neglect to use effective contraception, although pregnancy is most unwelcome. Family planning services are now available free on the National Health Service from general practitioners, or from local clinics for those who prefer these. Hospitals should advise their own obstetric and gynaecological patients, and also those with special medical or psychiatric problems.

It is important that doctors should have knowledge of all the available methods, and their advantages and disadvantages. After the initial consultation to choose the best method for the patient she must be followed up, and she should attend for a check at 3 months, and then regularly every 6 to 12 months, depending on the method. At each visit her blood pressure and weight are recorded, and cervical smears are taken at appropriate intervals.

Methods of contraception include:

1. Systemic contraception, using hormonal preparations:
   a. Oral contraceptives
      i. Combined pill, containing oestrogen and a progestogen.
      ii. Progestogen-only pill.
   b. Injectable contraceptives.
   c. Implants.
   d. Vaginal ring contraception.
   e. Postcoital contraception.
2. Intrauterine contraceptive devices, including those releasing
   a. Copper ions.
   b. Progestogen.
3. Methods that prevent access of sperm to the upper female genital tract:
   a. Vaginal cap or sponge, with spermicide.
   b. Condom.
   c. Coitus interruptus.
   d. Safe period.
4. Permanent methods — sterilization.

Failure rates

Methods of contraception vary in effectiveness. Reported failure rates vary widely according to the motivation of the patients and the care and training of their advisers. Table 23.1 is only for illustration:

ORAL CONTRACEPTION

This is a very effective method, provided that the patient takes the tablets correctly. Two types of pill are used: (1) combined pill, and (2) progestogen-only pill.

Table 23.1 Failure rates for contraceptive methods and for sterilization

Method	Number of unwanted pregnancies in 100 fertile women using the method for 1 year (Pearl index)
Sterilization (male or female)	0.1
Combined pill	0.1
Progestogen-only pill	2
Intrauterine device	1
Diaphragm with spermicide	6
Condom with spermicide	8
Coitus interruptus	20

The combined pill

This is the usual type. It contains both an oestrogen (usually ethinyl oestradiol) and a progestogen (see Table 23.2). Since the introduction of oral contraceptives 30 years ago the dose of oestrogen has been progressively reduced from 100 to 30 micrograms daily in the hope or reducing side-effects (see p. 337). However, with the present low-dose pills the margin of error is less, and correct tablet-taking is essential to avoid failure.

Method of action

The combined pill inhibits ovulation and makes cervical mucus more viscid, thus preventing penetration by sperm. There are also endometrial changes, so that if ovulation should occur implantation would be difficult. Because the endometrium is thinner, menstrual blood loss is reduced.

Formulations

In each cycle a pill is taken daily for 21 days and an interval of 7 days follows, during which a withdrawal bleed occurs.

Table 23.2 Examples of combined pills

	Oestrogen (micrograms)		Progestogen (micrograms)	
Monophasic				
Minovlar	Ethinyl oestradiol	50	Norethisterone acetate	1000
Eugynon 50	Ethinyl oestradiol	50	Levonorgestrel	250
Eugynon 30	Ethinyl oestradiol	30	Levonorgestrel	250
Microgynon	Ethinyl oestradiol	30	Levonorgestrel	150
Marvelon	Ethinyl oestradiol	30	Desogestrel	150
Norimin	Ethinyl oestradiol	35	Norethisterone	1000
Brevinor	Ethinyl oestradiol	35	Norethisterone	500
Biphasic				
Binovum 7 days	Ethinyl oestradiol	35	Norethisterone	500
14 days	Ethinyl oestradiol	35	Norethisterone	1000
Triphasic				
Trinovum 7 days	Ethinyl oestradiol	35	Norethisterone	500
7 days	Ethinyl oestradiol	35	Norethisterone	750
7 days	Ethinyl oestradiol	35	Norethisterone	1000
Trinordial 6 days	Ethinyl oestradiol	30	Levonorgestrel	50
5 days	Ethinyl oestradiol	40	Levonorgestrel	75
10 days	Ethinyl oestradiol	30	Levonorgestrel	125

The first cycle of pills is started on the first day of menstruation, to obtain maximum suppression of the pituitary, and to prevent breakthrough ovulation. In subsequent cycles, if bleeding does not occur during the pill-free days, then the next pack of pills is started after the 7-day gap. In the unlikely event of two 'periods' being missed the patient should be examined clinically and have an ultrasound scan or a pregnancy test.

Many preparations are available (see Table 23.2). Those mentioned are only named as examples, and there are many other preparations of equal merit. Monophasic pills contain a fixed daily dose of oestrogen and progestogen. Packs of biphasic pills are made up so that the dose of progestogen is varied once during the cycle, and in triphasic pills the dose of both oestrogen and progestogen may be varied twice. The purpose is to reduce the total dose of steroid and diminish side-effects.

Side-effects and complications

Important complications

1. Hypertension may occur, especially during the first year of use and in women over 35. It is less common with low-dose oestrogen pills and tri- or bi-phasic pills. The pressure must be recorded at each visit to the doctor or clinic. If the pressure rises an alternative method of contraception, such as the progestogen-only pill, must be used.
2. Thrombosis and vascular disease are slightly more common in pill users, especially in women over 35, and those who are overweight or smoke heavily. Combined oral contraceptives are not advised for any woman with a history of thrombosis or embolism, but uncomplicated varicose veins are not a contraindication. Provided that an alternative method of contraception is provided, the pill should be discontinued before any surgical procedure which carries a significant risk of thrombosis.

    Venous thrombosis and pulmonary embolism result from oestrogen-induced reduction of antithrombin in the blood, and are less common with low-oestrogen pills. In causing arterial disease, myocardial infarction and stroke, all of which are rare, both oestrogen and progestogens are implicated, but these complications are avoided with multiphasic and low-dose pills.
3. Cholestatic jaundice, similar to that sometimes seen during pregnancy, may occur. Recovery is rapid if the pills are stopped, but oral contraception is not advised for any patient with hepatic disease.
4. If a woman has an oestrogen-dependent tumour, such as breast cancer, pills containing oestrogen are contraindicated.

5. The first period after stopping oral contraception is often delayed. More persistent amenorrhoea is uncommon, and usually recovers spontaneously. It is more common in women who previously had irregular cycles.

Other side-effects

1. The oestrogen may cause nausea in the first cycle. If it persists the patient is examined to exclude pregnancy, and a change is made to a pill containing less oestrogen.
2. Tenderness and slight enlargement of the breasts may occur.
3. The 'menstrual' loss is usually reduced. Intermenstrual breakthrough bleeding may occur. If this persists it is usually controlled by changing the progestogen or increasing the dose of it.
4. An initial gain of weight of 0.5 kg is common. This is usually lost after a few cycles.
5. Cervical erosions are common.
6. Vaginal candidiasis may occur.
7. Facial pigmentation like that sometimes seen during pregnancy (choasma) rarely occurs.
8. Migrainous headaches may occur.
9. Psychological effects are difficult to assess. Depression is sometimes attributed to the pill, but seldom with much evidence. Fear of the pill is common because of unbalanced reports of its risks in the media.

Despite this long list of possible side-effects it should be realized that millions of women throughout the world are using the pill without any trouble.

Drug interaction

Certain drugs may reduce the effectiveness of contraceptive steroids. Unexplained intermenstrual bleeding may be the first sign of drug interaction.

Barbiturates, dichloralphenazone (Welldorm), phenytoin, rifampicin and griseofulvin may increase the activity of hepatic enzymes which metabolize steroids. Wide-spectrum antibiotics may interfere with the absorption of oestrogens from the gut.

Progestogen-only pill

These pills, which contain no oestrogen, are taken daily and continuously. They were introduced to avoid the side-effects of oestrogens.

Method of action

This type of pill increases the viscosity of cervical mucus and inhibits sperm penetration. In addition, in many women either normal ovulation does not occur or the luteal phase is abnormal, so that the endometrium is unreceptive.

The regime is simple for the patient, but the failure rate is slightly higher than for the combined pill. These pills are suitable for the older woman, and for those in whom oestrogens are contraindicated. They have the disadvantage that irregular endometrial bleeing sometimes occurs.

Examples of these pills are Micronor, containing 350 micrograms of norethisterone; Neogest, containing 35 micrograms of levonorgestrel; and Femulen, containing 500 micrograms of ethynodiol acetate.

Injectable contraceptives

Slow-release preparations of progestogens may be injected intramuscularly. Medroxyprogesterone acetate (Depo-Provera) 150 mg every 10 weeks or norethisterone oenanthate 200 mg, injected every 10 weeks. Both have the disadvantage that they may cause irregular bleeding, and once injected their effects are irreversible.

Implants

Levonorgestrel rods can be implanted in the inner aspect of the arm under local anaesthesia to obtain slow continuous release of progestogen for as long as 5 years.

Vaginal ring contraception

A silastic ring impregnated with oestrogen and progestogen, or with progestogen alone, is placed in the upper vagina. It is left there for 21 days and then removed for 7 days, during which withdrawal bleeding will occur. The ring causes no coital difficulties.

Postcoital contraception

Hormonal contraception given within 72 hours of unprotected intercourse, or after such an accident as a torn condom, can prevent pregnancy. One method is to give two combined pills, each containing ethinyl oestradiol 50 micrograms and norgestrel 250 micrograms, and to repeat this 12 hours later.

If the patient does not seek advice until more than 72 hours have elapsed an intrauterine contraceptive device (described below) can be inserted, and is effective up to 5 days after ovulation.

INTRAUTERINE CONTRACEPTIVE DEVICES

Inert silastic intrauterine devices were developed in the 1960s and have been widely used. Various shapes were designed to be straightened or compressed for insertion through a cannula into the uterus, without anaesthesia. Most devices have a thread attached which projects through the cervix, so that the presence of the device can be checked, and with which it can be removed. The action of the original devices was mechanical, by interfering with the embedding of the ovum. More recently medicated devices, which release copper ions or hormones, have come into use.

Copper-medicated devices

The Copper-7 (Gravigard), Copper-T and Multiload devices (see Fig. 23.1) all have fine copper wire wound round the stem. The copper ions which are released modify the concentration of trace elements in the endometrium and cervical mucus. Effective contraceptive action persists for up to 5 years, but continuous erosion may eventually lead to fragmentation of the wire.

Hormone-releasing devices

Another type of medicated device carries levonorgestrel in a porous cylinder around the stem, and releases 2 micrograms of hormone per day for up to 5 years. Such devices reduce

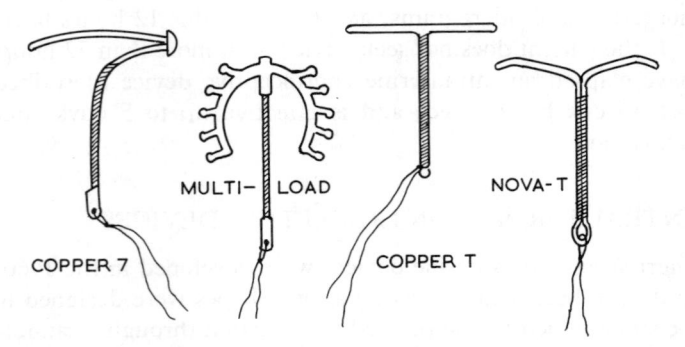

Fig. 23.1 Intrauterine devices.

the thickness of the endometrium and the amount of bleeding from it.

Method of insertion

Intrauterine devices should be inserted during menstruation when the cervix is relaxed. They can also be inserted immediately after miscarriage or termination of pregnancy, or soon after delivery. Before insertion the uterine position is checked by vaginal examination. A speculum is passed and the device is inserted into the uterus with an introducer, which leaves the device in place when it is withdrawn. The patient should be seen again after her next period, and then 6-monthly.

Selection of patients

Intrauterine devices are best used for family spacing in multiparous patients. They are contraindicated if there is any suspicion of pelvic infection. Because of the slight possibility of pelvic infection which might damage the tubes, the method is not recommended for nulliparae.

Side-effects

Intrauterine devices act on the endometrium and not on the Fallopian tubes, and ectopic pregnancy may sometimes occur.

All devices may cause minor intermenstrual bleeding and, except with the levonorgestrel device, periods may be heavier and last longer, but patients usually tolerate this. In a few cases there is colicky pain and more severe bleeding, necessitating removal of the device.

The risk of pelvic infection has already been mentioned.

A device may be expelled by uterine contractions, usually in the first 6 months of use.

Occasionally during insertion the uterus is perforated, and

the device enters the peritoneal cavity. If this is suspected, the threads of the device will not be seen, and ultrasound will show its position. If it is in the peritoneal cavity it must be removed, usually by laparoscopy.

If pregnancy occurs with an intrauterine device in place it is removed if traction on the threads brings it away easily, as this may reduce the risk of abortion. Otherwise it is left, and sometimes pregnancy continues uneventfully, and the device is delivered with the placenta.

METHODS PREVENTING ACCESS OF SPERM

Vaginal diaphragm with spermicide

The 'Dutch cap' is a soft rubber diaphragm with a thickened rim. The rim fits the vaginal vault obliquely so that the diaphragm covers the cervix. The commonest size required is 75 mm in diameter. Spermicidal cream is placed on both aspects of the diaphragm before insertion, and it is left in place for six hours after intercourse. The patient must be taught how to insert the cap correctly.

Condom (male sheath)

Because it is easy to buy, and no professional advice is required, the condom is still widely used. A spermicidal lubricant increases security against displacement or tearing of the sheath. The condom gives some protection against sexually transmitted disease.

Spermicidal sponge

Used alone, spermicides are unreliable. Recently a disposable sponge impregnated with a spermicide (Nonoxyl-9) has been introduced. The sponge acts as a partial barrier and increases the concentration of spermicide near the cervix.

Coitus interruptus

By this is meant withdrawal of the penis just before ejaculation. Although it is widely practised it is an unreliable method, probably because it is not well managed.

Safe period

At present this is the only method permitted to strict Roman Catholics. Intercourse is avoided for 3 days before and 2 days after the date of ovulation. Since the length of the cycle varies and the date of ovulation in any cycle is uncertain, this is a most unreliable method, even if a basal temperature chart is kept.

PERMANENT METHODS — STERILIZATION

Although attempts have been made to devise reversible methods of sterilization these have had little success, and couples should be told that for practical purposes this method of contraception is permanent, and is therefore only suitable for those with completed families or medical contraindications to pregnancy. Before sterilization of either partner it is essential to obtain detailed social and medical histories, and to find out the reasons for preferring sterilization to contraception. The written consent of both partners should be recorded.

Full information about methods and risks must be given. The decision must not be hurried. In general, unless the couple have been considering sterilization for some time, it is unwise to perform puerperal or postabortal sterilization, as regret and guilt feelings, and marital difficulties, may follow hasty decision. Sterilization should not be advised in cases of marital disharmony. A few young couples under 30 years of age will request sterilization; they require most careful counselling and for them a method which is at least potentially reversible, such as the use of clips, may be chosen.

Female sterilization

The following methods may be mentioned. General anaesthesia is usual, although local or regional anaesthesia is possible.

1. *Tubal ligation.* Through a very small abdominal incision ('mini-laparotomy') the proximal parts of both tubes are excised, and the cut ends are tied.
2. *Tubal diathermy.* Through a laparoscope about 2 cm of each tube is coagulated. The method carries risks in inexperienced hands as other structures may be injured. To avoid the risks of intraperitoneal diathermy the following methods are now preferred:
3. *Falope rings.* Using a laparoscope a 3 cm loop of the proximal part of each tube is drawn into the grip of a tight silastic ring. This causes necrosis of the loop and blockage of the ends.
4. *Tubal clips.* With a laparoscope a clip is applied to each tube. The Filshie titanium clip has a silastic insert which maintains occlusive pressure. The simplicity of this method commends it.

Failure and complications

Sterilization occasionally fails, usually within 18 months of the operation. For medico-legal reasons patients should always be warned of this possibility. A subsequent pregnancy is more likely to be ectopic than uterine.

After sterilization there may be alteration in the menstrual cycle, but this is usually a reflection of previous contraceptive practice; the woman's cycle reverts to that which she had before starting the contraceptive method. There is no good statistical evidence of an increased incidence of dysfunctional bleeding, dysmenorrhoea or fibromyomata after sterilization.

Reversal of sterilization is occasionally requested. With

modern microsurgery tubal patency may sometimes be re-established if the tubes have not been extensively damaged.

Male sterilization

Vasectomy is performed under local anaesthesia. Through a small scrotal incision on each side the vas deferens is identified, and after excising a small section both ends are doubly ligatured. It is not immediately effective as sperm remain for a time in the seminal vesicles. Until two specimens, taken at 3 and 4 months after the operation, have been shown to contain no sperms, some other method of contraception must be continued.

TERMINATION OF PREGNANCY

Termination of pregnancy before the child is viable involves difficult ethical decisions. Some believe that the killing of a fetus does not differ in principle from the murder of a baby, whereas others hold that a woman should not be forced to continue an unwanted pregnancy. No method of termination is without some risk to life, health or fertility — and contraception is a much better method of avoiding unwanted pregnancy.

In Britain the Abortion Act (1967) permits termination of pregnancy if its continuance would involve risk (greater than that of termination):

1. To the patient's life.
2. To her physical or mental health.
3. To the physical or mental health of the existing child(ren) 'of her family'.
4. Pregnancy may also be terminated if there is 'substantial risk' that the child will have such physical or mental abnormalities that it will be 'seriously handicapped'.

Careful discussion, without pressure on or direction of the patient, is essential before any decision.

A certificate must be signed by two doctors, neither of whom need necessarily be the doctor who performs the operation. The operator must notify the Department of Health that he has terminated the pregnancy. The operation must be performed in an NHS hospital or a place approved by the Department. A doctor or nurse who has conscientious objections is not required to act.

The purely medical indications for induction of abortion are seldom absolute. Such conditions as nephritis which is progressing, malignant hypertension, diabetes with renal or retinal disease, carcinoma of the breast, and serious cases of mental disease are rare. The majority of terminations are performed for combined medical and social reasons.

Fetal indications for termination have included rubella and some inherited diseases, certain of which can be diagnosed by amniocentesis.

Methods

1. *Vaginal evacuation.* The best method is to aspirate the uterine contents with a suction curette. Before the 8th week a small plastic Karman catheter can be used with minimal cervical dilatation and only local paracervical anaesthesia.

   From 8 to 12 weeks general anaesthesia and cervical dilatation are required before aspiration with a larger cannula. This method is dangerous after the 12th week. The later the termination the greater are the risks of incomplete evacuation, cervical damage, haemorrhage and sepsis.
2. *Prostaglandins.* Various synthetic esters of PGE_2 are available as vaginal pessaries, and are effective in inducing abortion.

3. *Intra-amniotic injections.* Injection of a concentrated solution of urea (80 g in 200 ml of water) into the amniotic cavity by the abdominal route usually causes abortion. Urea is preferable to hypertonic saline, which may cause sloughing if it is accidentally injected into the tissues or peritoneal cavity, or electrolytic disturbance if it enters a vein.
4. *Abdominal hysterotomy* may be required if other methods fail. It has the risks of laparotomy and leaves a uterine scar.

   Sterilization by tubal ligature or excision can be performed at the time of hysterotomy, but after vaginal termination sterilization is performed by a laparascopic technique.

After spontaneous abortion or termination of pregnancy an intramuscular injection of 100 micrograms of anti-D gamma globulin should be given if the patient is rhesus negative.

24

Backache in women

A *woman with backache usually has something wrong with her back*. In relatively few cases is a visceral cause found. A patient whose backache is caused by a gynaecological disorder has additional gynaecological symptoms, or else definite pelvic physical signs. Pain referred from the pelvic organs is not felt higher up than the lower lumbar region. If movements of the back are limited or painful there is a local cause.

Gynaecological causes of backache include:

1. Prolapse (occasionally).
2. Retroversion seldom causes backache; it is possible in cases with prolapse or with infection.
3. Inflammatory lesions such as cervicitis or salpingitis.
4. Malignant metastases.

Postural defects and muscular weakness are common causes of backache in the puerperium. Rarely, sacro-iliac strain, symphysial separation or coccygeal fracture follow delivery, and a prolapsed intervertebral disc may date from that time.

The other multitudinous causes of backache will not be described, but may be broadly classified into:

1. Referred pain from the renal tract, from other viscera, or from lesions of the spinal cord (rare).
2. Pain due to local lesions of bones, joints, ligaments, muscles or fasciae (common).

25

Urinary disorders in gynaecological patients

FREQUENCY OF MICTURITION AND DYSURIA

Causes of frequency and discomfort on micturition related to gynaecology include:

1. *Urethral lesions*: gonococcal and non-specific (chlamydial) urethritis. Traumatic urethritis ('honeymoon cystitis'). Urethral caruncle (p. 262). Urethral diverticulum (p. 262).
2. *Cystitis* following catheterization, pelvic operations or irradiation. With cystocele.
3. *Pressure on the bladder* from the pregnant uterus or a pelvic tumour.

URINARY INCONTINENCE

True incontinence may be active (e.g. nocturnal enuresis) or passive (e.g. leak from a fistula, or sphincter paralysis from a neurological disorder). *False (overflow) incontinence* may occur in cases of long-standing retention from any cause, when urine dribbles from the overdistended bladder past the obstruction.

Fistulae

Vesicovaginal fistula (see p. 228)

Ureteric fistula

The ureter may be cut or tied during a pelvic operation, or it may slough because of impaired blood supply after dissection in Wertheim's hysterectomy. Half of the total output of urine escapes into the vaginal vault through the fistula. A pyelogram will show a dilated ureter above the fistulous track. Repair is seldom possible, and reimplantation into the bladder is usually required. If ureteric obstruction is unrelieved a pyonephrosis may form, or the kidney may atrophy.

In gynaecological practice *partial incontinence* is more often encountered. As many as 5% of young nulliparae and about 20% of older parous women have occasional incontinence which is sufficient to be an inconvenience. Two forms occur:

Stress incontinence

In this disorder the detrusor activity of the bladder is normal, but sphincter function is impaired. Involuntary escape of urine occurs when the intra-abdominal pressure is suddenly raised for example on coughing, or during heavy exertion. Stress incontinence is usually the result of damage to the region of the bladder neck during delivery, but it may also be seen in elderly women. Although it may be associated with cystocele it is a separate lesion.

Urge incontinence

In this condition the sphincter mechanism is normal, but the bladder is overactive. The involuntary escape of urine is associated with a desire to void. It may be subdivided into motor urge incontinence, in which there are uninhibited detrusor contractions, and sensory urge incontinence, in which there is heightened bladder sensitivity to filling. The overactivity may result from a local irritative lesion such as cystitis, but in many cases no cause is evident.

Physiology of continence

There is some uncertainty about the precise mechanism of bladder control in the female. Radiological studies show that, except during voiding, urethral closure is maintained by the compressor urethrae muscle, assisted by *striped* muscle fibres in the wall of the urethra.

Fibres from the medial edge of levator ani are also inserted into the urethra, and normally produce an angle between the base of the bladder and the posterior wall of the urethra. When the woman voids this angle opens out. However, this is a subsidiary rather than an essential mechanism in maintaining continence.

If the bladder neck is in the normal position and the abdominal pressure rises sharply, some of the pressure is exerted on the part of the urethra above the pelvic diaphragm and tends to close it (Fig. 25.1). If the opening in the pelvic diaphragm is stretched and the bladder neck descends, there is loss of this lateral pressure on the uretha.

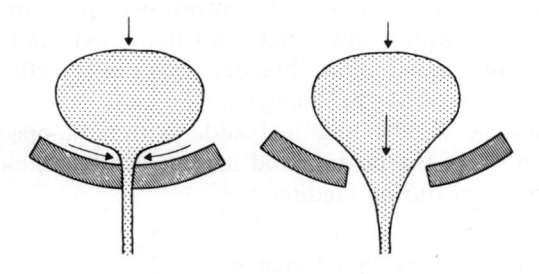

Fig. 25.1 Diagrams to show bladder neck. Normally any increase in intra-abdominal pressure tends to close the urethra. With descent of the bladder neck this protection is lost.

In all cases of partial incontinence careful assessment is required. Any infection which may cause bladder irritation must be treated. Distinction between urge incontinence and stress incontinence is very important, because surgical treatment will not help the former.

Investigation

Examination may include:

1. *Direct observation of any leak of urine* on coughing. Obviously for this the bladder must not be empty. If there is uncertainty about the degree of incontinence the patient is asked to wear a vulval pad during 30 minutes of active exercise. Weighing the pad before and afterwards will indicate the urinary loss.
2. *Cystometry.* Fluid is slowly infused into the bladder through a catheter. A continuous recording is made of the volume of fluid in the bladder and the intravesical pressure. A second fluid-filled catheter leading to a small balloon is placed in the rectum to measure the intra-abdominal pressure. Subtraction of the intra-abdominal pressure from the intravesical pressure gives the pressure caused by detrusor activity. During voiding the rate of urinary flow relative to the intravesical pressure can be measured with a flowmeter, and if the patient is told to stop voiding before the bladder is empty the efficiency of the sphincter can be assesssed.
3. *Radiology.* After filling the bladder with radio-opaque fluid the form of the bladder and urethra can be studied, both at rest and during voiding.

Treatment of urge incontinence

It has to be said that the treatment of urge incontinence is often ineffective. Some relief can be obtained with mild tranquillizing drugs such as Impramine, and anticholinergic drugs such as emepromium bromide (Ceteprim 200 mg three times daily) may reduce detrusor activity. Success has followed bladder training in hospital, in which the patient is taught to hold back her visits to the lavatory at progressively longer intervals.

Treatment of stress incontinence

In the early weeks after delivery improvement may be gained from pelvic floor exercises under the supervision of a physiotherapist, but most patients eventually require surgical treatment. The aim is to elevate the bladder neck so that the upper urethra is restored to the position where the intra-abdominal pressure can act upon it, and also to tighten the fascial structures around the urethra. If there is a cystocele anterior colporrhaphy (p. 360) is performed, and this will relieve more than half of the patients. For those with no cystocele, or in whom colporrhaphy has not cured the incontinence, abdominal procedures are often recommended.

In the Marshall–Marchetti–Krantz operation a suprapubic incision is made, and the anterior wall of the bladder is drawn up and then stitched to the fascia on the posterior aspect of the pubic bone and the abdominal wall. The Burch operation is a more recent modification of this, in which the fascia posterior and lateral to the bladder neck is drawn up and sutured to the iliopectineal ligament on each side.

There is also a place for sling operations such as that of Aldridge. In a modern variant of it a silastic sling is fixed above to the aponeurosis of the external oblique muscle and drawn down behind the symphysis pubis so as to surround, elevate and constrict the upper urethra.

RETENTION OF URINE

In women retention of urine may be caused by:

1. Pelvic tumours, including a retroverted gravid uterus, a fibromyoma or an ovarian tumour. Haematocolpos, pelvic haematocele or pelvic abscess are rare causes.
2. Procidentia, occasionally.
3. Postoperative or puerperal bruising of the bladder neck.
4. Extradural anaesthesia, or division of the pelvic nerve plexuses at Wertheim's hysterectomy. In both cases gradual recovery of bladder tone usually occurs.
5. Hysteria, and neurological disorders such as multiple sclerosis and spinal cord injury.

26

Notes on gynaecological operations

Details of surgical technique hardly concern the student, but a few general notes about gynaecological operations may be useful.

The date chosen for operation may need to be related to the menstrual cycle (e.g. for endometrial biopsy). Repair operations may be postponed if a period is due, but this is unimportant for hysterectomy or for minor procedures. If the patient is using an oral contraceptive containing oestrogen this should be discontinued before any major procedure because of the risk of thrombosis, but an alternative must be provided during any waiting period.

The patient should be admitted at least 2 days before a major operation. Many minor procedures are performed as day-cases, but sufficient time must always be allowed for preoperative examination with special attention to oral sepsis, anaemia, the circulation and the lungs. The urine is tested for protein and glucose, and a midstream specimen is often required for bacteriological examination. Anaemic patients may require blood transfusion.

The rectum should be empty before major procedures; if necessary a laxative or simple enema is given. The bladder must also be empty, and the safest plan is to pass a catheter in the theatre.

Before abdominal section the skin is purified in the usual way. Before vaginal operations any evident local infection is treated, and oestrogens may be given to an elderly patient if there is atrophic vaginitis. The vulva is shaved, but vaginal douching is a waste of time, and painting the vagina with an antiseptic solution can only be done effectively with the patient anaesthetized. Many surgeons give oral metronidazole before major procedures.

Vaginal and perineal operations

These are performed with the patient in the lithotomy position.

Dilatation of the cervix and curettage

A vaginal speculum is inserted and the cervix is held with a volsellum. The uterine sound is passed, followed by a graduated series of cervical dilators, before the curette is used. Ring forceps may be useful to seize a polyp. Complications: cervical incompetence, perforation of the uterus.

Endometrial biopsy can also be performed with a suction curette such as the Vabra aspirator without anaesthesia. It is not certain that this is as reliable as curettage for investigation of possible malignant disease.

Operation to enlarge the vaginal orifice

An incision is made along the posterior margin of the orifice and a flap of vaginal epithelium is raised from the underlying perineal body. After incising the perineal body in the midline to enlarge the orifice the epithelial flap is sutured back to cover the raw area.

Amputation of the cervix

Not often done, except as part of the Manchester operation

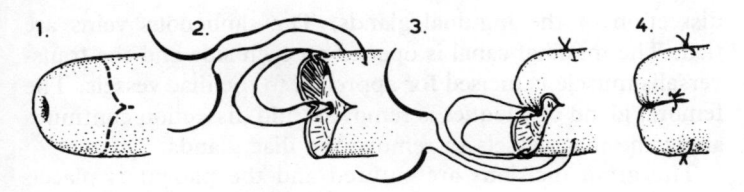

Fig. 26.1 Amputation of cervix.

(see below). Figure 26.1 shows the method. Secondary haemorrhage is an occasional complication, and is treated with a vaginal gauze pack.

Cervical cauterization, cryosurgery and laser coagulation
See p. 276.

Radical excision of the vulva

With the patient in the dorsal position an oblique incision is made in each groin and flaps are undermined to allow block

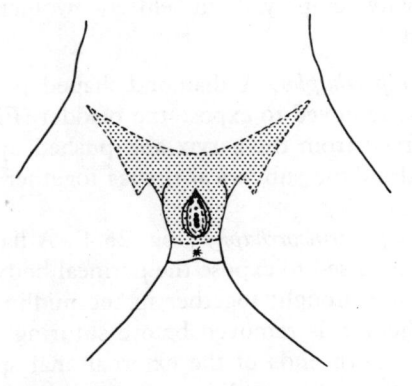

Fig. 26.2 Radical excision of vulva.

dissection of the inguinal glands. The saphenous veins are tied. The inguinal canal is opened on each side and the transversalis muscle is incised for approach to the iliac vessels. The femoral gland of Cloquet is removed, and dissection continues along the iliac vessels to remove the iliac glands.

The groin incisions are sutured and the patient is placed in the lithotomy position. The vulva is excised by the incision shown. It is often impossible to close the raw area completely and it is left to granulate. A self-retaining catheter is inserted, and the wound is kept dry until it granulates, when bathing can start.

Operations for prolapse

The choice of operation may be:

1. For cystocele: anterior colporrhaphy.
2. For rectocele and deficient perineum: posterior colpoperineorrhaphy.
3. For uterine descent (usually there is also cystocele and rectocele): Manchester (Fothergill) operation, or vaginal hysterectomy, with anterior and posterior colporrhaphy.
4. Occasionally employed in elderly women: Le Fort's operation.

Anterior colporrhaphy. A diamond-shaped piece of vaginal epithelium is removed to expose the bladder (Fig. 26.3). The bladder is freed from the cervix and pushed up. Sutures are inserted to draw the subvesical tissues together and close the diamond.

Posterior colpoperineorrhaphy (Fig. 26.4). A flap of posterior vaginal wall is raised to expose the perineal body. The levator ani muscles are brought together in the midline. Redundant vaginal epithelium is removed before suturing. If the tear is complete, the torn ends of the external anal sphincter must be freed and brought together.

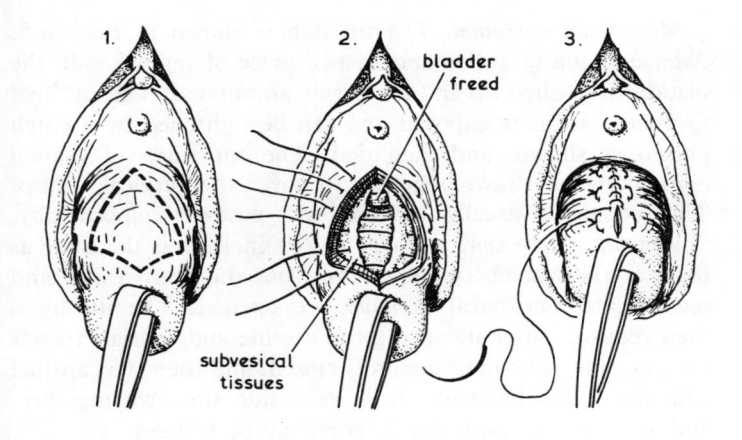

Fig. 26.3 Diagram to show principle of anterior colporrhaphy.

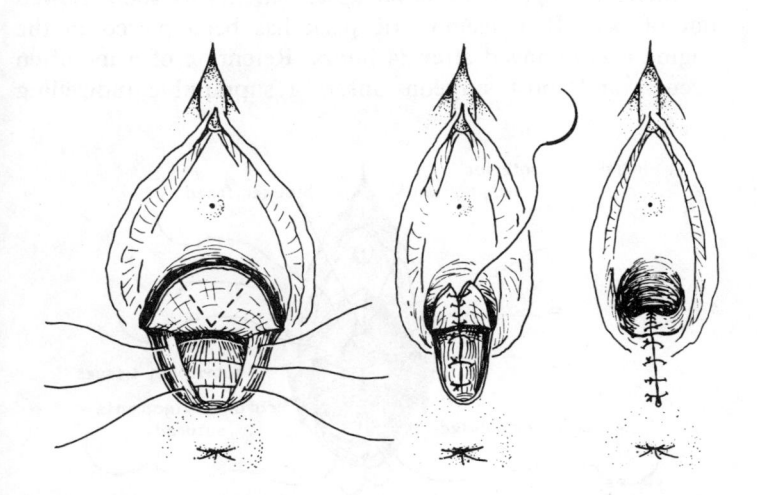

Fig. 26.4 Diagram to show stages of posterior colpoperineorrhaphy.

Manchester operation. The incision is shown in Fig. 26.5. After excision of a diamond-shaped piece of vaginal wall, the bladder is pushed up and the cervix amputated. The cardinal ligaments are now exposed and can be tightened by a stitch passed as shown, and then tied. The cut edges of vaginal epithelium are drawn together to cover the cervical stump. The operation is usually combined with posterior colporrhaphy.

Vaginal hysterectomy and repair. The incision is the same as that for the Manchester operation, but the uterovesical and rectovaginal peritoneal pouches are opened. The uterus is then removed after ligaturing the uterine and ovarian vessels on each side. The peritoneum is closed, and then the cardinal and uterosacral ligaments from each side are sewn together, and anterior and posterior colporrhapy performed.

Le Fort's operation. A strip is excised from the anterior vaginal wall, and a similar strip from the posterior wall, and the two raw areas are sewn together to form a vaginal septum.

Aftercare of operations for prolapse. Patients are soon allowed out of bed. If a haemostatic pack has been placed in the vagina it is removed after 24 hours. Retention of urine often occurs, and most surgeons insert a suprapubic indwelling

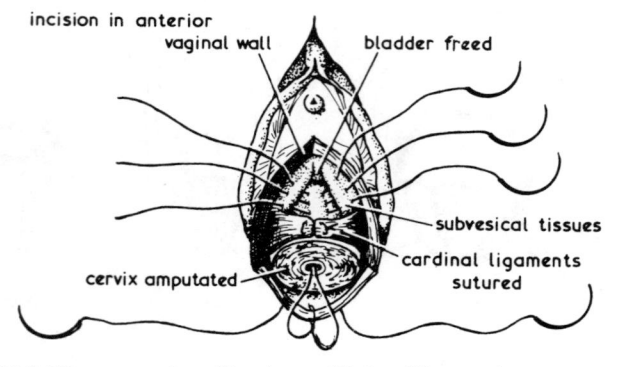

Fig. 26.5 Diagram to show Manchester (Fothergill) operation.

catheter for 2 to 5 days. Antibiotics may be required for urinary infection. The perineum is kept as dry as possible, and douching is best avoided. Absorbable stitches do not require removal, but a vaginal examination is made on the 10th day, when any abnormal adhesions are easily broken down with the finger. Care is taken not to narrow the vagina unduly if intercourse is still practised.

If the anal sphincter has been repaired the bowel is confined for 4 days, then opened with a small enema after instillation of olive oil to soften the faeces. In other cases an aperient is given on the 3rd day, and an enema subsequently if necessary.

Shock is unusual even in elderly patients. Secondary haemorrhage from a vessel at the vaginal vault can be controlled with a gauze pack. Retention of urine and cystitis are common. Minor local sepsis usually resolves.

Operations for stress incontinence

See p. 355.

Abdominal operations

These are often performed with the patient in the Trendelenburg (head-down) position to allow the intestines to fall away from the pelvis. Apart from the ordinary paramedian or midline incisions, a low transverse incision is commonly used.

Aftercare and complications. Early deep breathing and leg movements are important. Patients are usually out of bed on the first day, but are likely to be in hospital for 14 days. An aperient may be given on about the 4th day, or a simple enema.

Complications such as those of any laparotomy, including anaesthetic problems, ileus, wound haematoma or sepsis, wound dehiscence and incisional hernia are treated in the usual way. The following complications may merit special mention:

Retention of urine. If this does not respond to carbachol 250 micrograms intramuscularly, catheterization is required.

Dangerous intraperitoneal haemorrhage can occur from a slipped ligature on the ovarian or uterine artery, and call for urgent laparotomy. Secondary haemorrhage from sepsis in the vaginal vault is controlled with a gauze pack.

Femoral thrombosis and pulmonary embolism may follow thrombosis which starts in the veins of the calf and spreads upwards. Pressure on the calf on the operating table, and subsequent lack of movement, are predisposing factors. In a few gynaecological cases primary thrombosis of pelvic veins occurs, when operative trauma or pelvic sepsis are contributory factors. Blood coagulability and the platelet count rise to a maximum 7 to 10 days after injury or haemorrhage, which is a common time for thrombosis to occur. Some surgeons use prophylactic measures for all major operations: (1) intravenous infusions of dextran can be given to reduce platelet adhesiveness, (2) small doses of heparin can be given by subcutaneous injection, or (3) a simple and risk-free method is to encase the legs in plastic bags in which the pressure can be varied intermittently during the operation to increase the venous flow.

In cases with calf pain or swelling anticoagulants are used. Heparin 10 000 units is given intravenously 4-hourly for 48 hours. Warfarin 50 mg is given orally on the first day. The prothrombin time is estimated on the 3rd day, and then treatment is continued with doses of 3 to 10 mg daily according to the effect on the prothrombin activity of the blood.

Hysterectomy

Hysterectomy may be by the vaginal or the abdominal route.

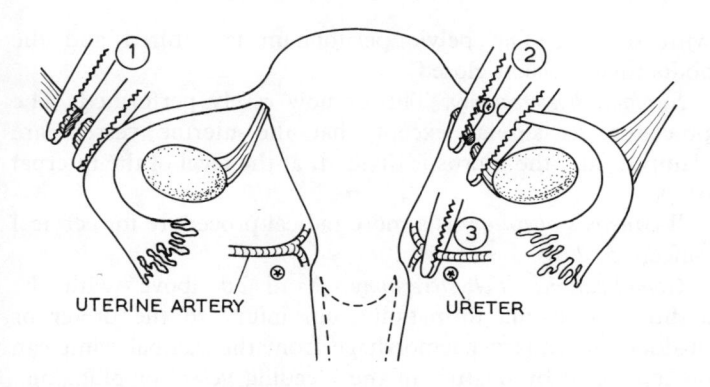

Fig. 26.6 Diagram to show position of clamps in hysterectomy: (1) division of infundibulo-pelvic ligament containing ovarian vessels, lateral to the ovary and tube, if these are to be removed with the uterus; (2) division of broad ligament and ovarian vessels medial to the ovary if the ovary is to be retained; (3) clamp on uterine vessels (the proximity of the ureter has been exaggerated).

In total abdominal hysterectomy the whole uterus is removed; in subtotal hysterectomy the cervix is left. Especially in parous women, total hysterectomy is best, as the cervix is often unhealthy and might later be the site of carcinoma. Before the menopause, the ovaries, or part of an ovary, are conserved whenever possible.

Total hysterectomy. After opening the abdomen the broad ligaments (containing the ovarian vessels) are divided between clamps. If the ovary is to be removed the infundibulo-pelvic ligament is divided, otherwise the broad ligament is divided medially to the ovary. The peritoneum of the utero-vesical pouch is incised transversely, and the bladder is freed from the front of the cervix. The uterine vessels are clamped and divided close to the cervix, avoiding the ureter. After cutting around the vaginal vault the uterus is removed. Clamps on vessels are replaced by ligatures. The vaginal vault is closed with sutures. The pelvic peritoneum is sutured and the abdominal incision closed.

Subtotal hysterectomy. This is now rarely performed. The procedure is similar except that the uterine vessels are clamped, and the uterus is divided, at the level of the internal os.

Wertheim's operation is a more radical procedure for cervical cancer (p. 278).

Complications of hysterectomy. As listed above, with the addition of fistula formation from injury to the ureter or bladder. Secondary haemorrhage from the vaginal vault can be controlled by ligature of the bleeding vessel or plugging.

Abdominal myomectomy

Before enucleating fibromyomata some surgeons temporarily occlude the uterine vessels with a rubber-covered clamp that encircles the uterus at the level of the internal os, and also the ovarian vessels with a clamp on each infundibulo-pelvic ligament. After shelling-out the fibroids any cavities left in the uterine wall are obliterated with sutures.

The operation may fail in that fibroids may recur or sterility follow.

(A polypoid submucous fibroid can be removed by *vaginal myomectomy*, by division of the pedicle after drawing the tumour down with a volsellum.)

Ventrosuspension for retroversion

This is now seldom performed (see p. 235).

Operation for ovarian cysts and tumours

For large cysts it is better to make a long paramedian or midline incision and remove the cyst entire rather than to withdraw it through a small incision after tapping, which may disseminate malignant cells. If the tumour is free the pedicle is easily clamped and divided and ligatured by a transfixion suture. Adherent tumours such as endometriomata are similarly removed after freeing adhesions, which may be a far more difficult procedure.

Benign cysts may be enucleated from the thinned-out ovary, or partial oöphorectomy may be possible. Even a small portion of ovary is worth conserving in a young woman, but in women over 45 the opposite ovary is also removed if there is the least abnormality.

If an ovarian tumour is considered to be malignant, both tubes and ovaries and the uterus are removed.

The aftercare is as described above for any abdominal operation. There is a risk of an ovarian ligature slipping if the pedicle is not transfixed.

Broad ligament cysts are enucleated after incision of the peritoneum over them, taking care that the ureter is not pushed up and endangered.

Salpingectomy and salpingo-oöphorectomy

If the tube is to be removed for ectopic gestation clamps are placed on the mesosalpinx and at the uterine cornu. After excising the tube the clamps are replaced by ligatures.

Operations for salpingo-oöphoritis are far more difficult. Adhesions are gradually divided until tube and ovary are free, when the ovarian vessels are controlled by clamping the infundibulo-pelvic ligament. The tube and often the ovary are removed, any other vessels are tied, and raw surfaces are covered with peritoneum whenever possible.

Operations for tubal occlusion

See p. 326.

Sterilization

See p. 345.

'Presacral' neurectomy

See p. 314.

Other procedures for investigation

Colposcopy and cervical biopsy

See p. 273.

Laparoscopy

With general anaesthesia, the patient is placed in the dorsal position with Trendelenburg tilt and her legs separated with stirrups. After emptying the bladder and placing a cannula in the cervical canal, a needle is inserted through the abdominal wall. The peritoneal cavity is inflated with carbon dioxide, so that the intestines are displaced from the pelvis. An abdominal cannula is then inserted to carry the light system and telescope through which the pelvic organs are examined. A separate small cannula can be inserted to carry a biopsy drill, a diathermy electrode for sterilization by coagulating the tubes, or a device for putting clips on the tubes. Methylene blue solution can be injected through the cervical cannula; its escape will be seen if the tubes are patent. The patient can usually go home the next day.

This procedure requires both special training and skill. Injury to the bowel or other structures may otherwise occur, especially if diathermy is used. The inflation of the peritoneum may cause cardiac arrest, and the anaesthetist must use atropine and also intubate the trachea.

Hysteroscopy

Under general anaesthesia a small telescope is inserted through the cervix. The uterine cavity is distended with fluid (Dextran) or carbon dioxide gas. Such lesions as polypi, early carcinoma or intrauterine adhesions may then be seen. Benign lesions can be coagulated with a laser beam.

Index

Abdominal pregnancy, 70
Abortion, 63 et seq.
  induction of, 347 et seq.
  recurrent, 66
Abruptio placentae, 88 et seq.
Achondroplasia, 131
Acidosis, 49
Acromegaly, 304
Acroparaesthesia, 113
ACTH, 34, 227
Acute fevers, 105, 106
Adenomyosis, 298
Addison's disease, 305
Adrenal disorders, 305
Adrenogenital syndrome, 226, 303
AIDS, 241
Alcoholism, 114
Aldridge sling operation, 353
Alpha-fetoprotein, 28
Allantois, 217, 218
Amenorrhoea
  pregnancy of, 21
  primary, 220, 302
  secondary, 304
Amniocentesis, 186
Amnion, 19
Amniotic embolism, 153
Amniotic fluid, 19, 186
Amniotomy, 174
Amputation of cervix, 358
Anaemia in pregnancy, 98
  of newborn, 169

Anaesthesia, 118, 121, 124, 126, 140, 141, 144, 151
Analgesia, 117, 124
  epidural, 133, 180
Androblastoma, 289
Androgens, 7
Android pelvis, 130
Androstenedione, 7
Anencephaly, 26, 129
Angioma of placenta, 86
Anorexia nervosa, 305
Anovular cycles, 308
Anoxia, fetal, 49, 189
Antenatal care, 26 et seq.
Antenatal exercises, 31
Antepartum haemorrhage, 87 et seq.
Anthropoid pelvis, 130
Anticoagulants, 364
Anti D globulin, 171
Anuria, 83, 163
Aorta, coarctation, 101
Apgar score, 191
Appendicitis, 108
Areola, 22
Arrhenoblastoma, 289
Artificial feeding, 196
Artificial insemination
  donor sperm, 328
  husband's sperm, 328
Ascites, 258, 287, 289, 291
Asphyxia neonatorum, 189 et seq.

INDEX

Assimilation of sacrum, 131
Asthma, 103
Atelectasis, 192
Atrophic vaginitis, 247
Attitude, fetal, 29
Augmentation of labour, 47
Autosomes, 223
Azoospermia, 328

Backache, 350
Bacteraemic shock, 65
Bacteriuria, 83
Bacteroides, 156
Balottement, 23
Bandl's retraction ring, 137
Bartholin's glands, 237
    cyst, 261
    diseases of, 244
Basal body temperature, 322
Battledore placenta, 19
Bile ducts, atresia, 205
Bilirubin, 199, 204
Bimanual compression, 144
Birth injuries, 199
Bladder, hyperkinetic, 354
Botryoid sarcoma, uterus, 281
Brachial palsy, 201
Brandt-Andrews manoeuvre, 54
Breast, physiology, 22
    care of, 57
    feeding, 195
    neonatal engorgement, 160, 194
    puerperal abnormalities, 57, 160
Breech presentation, 121 et seq.
Bregma, 41
Brenner tumour, 288
Broad ligament, 230
    haematoma of,
    tumours of, 296
Bromocriptine, 304
Brow presentation, 120
Bruserelin, 329

Caesarean section, 181
    for breech, 125
    for disproportion, 131

Caesarean section scar, rupture, 185
Caesium, 276
Candidiasis, 246
Caput succedaneum, 40
Carcinoma in situ, cervix, 271, 274
Carcinoma in pregnancy, 97
Cardiac disease and pregnancy, 100
Cardinal ligament, 230
Cardiovascular side-effects oral contraception, 338
Carneous mole, 66
Carpal tunnel syndrome, 113
Caruncle, urethral, 262
Caudal anaesthesia, 180
Cellulitis, pelvic, 157
Cephalhaematoma, 40, 199
Cervix
    biopsy, 274
    carcinoma, 97, 271
    cervicitis, 247
    changes in pregnancy and labour, 22
    congenital abnormalities, 221
    cytology, 29
    discharge, 250
    dysplasia, 274
    dystocia, 137
    ectropion, 249
    erosion, 59, 249
    incompetence, 67
    injuries and lacerations, 149, 229
    intraepithelial neoplasia, 274
    operations, 359
    polyp, 270
    secretion of, 322
    stenosis, 134
Chancre, 239
Chancroid, 240
Chicken pox, 105
Chlamydia, 107, 238
Chloasma, 22
Chlorambucil, 295
Cholestatic jaundice with oral contraception, 338

Chorea gravidarum, 110
Choriocarcinoma, 68
Chorion, 19
  villi, 17, 18
Chorionic villus sampling, 187
Chromosomal analysis, 223
  abnormality, 220
Chronic nephritis, 82
Chronic salpingitis, 254
CIN classification, 274
Clear cell tumour, ovary, 287
Cleidotomy, 186
Clitoris, 218
Clomiphene citrate, 325
Clostridia, 156
Coagulation disorders, 146
Coarctation of aorta, 101
Coitus, 16
  transit of sperm
Coitus interruptus, 345
Coliform organisms, 156, 159
Colostrum, 22
Colpocleisis, 229
Colporrhapy,
  delivery after, 355
  operations, 361
Colposcopy, 250, 272
Combined pill (contraception), 336
Condom, 334
Condylomata
  vulval, 260
Congenital malformations of the
  fetus, 26, 28, 84, 86, 93, 95,
  113, 115, 128 et seq., 138
Conjugate
  diagonal, 37
  true, 37
Conjunctivitis, 206
Convelaire uterus, 88
Constriction ring, 136
Contraception, 333 et seq.
Convulsions, eclamptic, 77
  in new born, 207
Coomb's test, 171
Copper intrauterine devices, 342
Cord, *see* Umbilical cord

Corpus albicans, 5
Corpus luteum, 3, 17
Corticotrophin, 19
Cramps, 113
Craniotomy, 186
Cryoprobe, 250
Cryptomenorrhoea, 222
Cumulus oophorus, 5
Curettage, 358
Cushing's disease, 305
Cystic glandular hyperplasia, 309
Cystocoele, 233
Cystometry, 354
Cytology, vaginal
  cervical, 273
Cytomegalic virus, 107
Cytotoxic drugs, 295
Cytotrophoblast, 17

Danazol, 301
Decidua, 16
Deep transverse arrest, 116
Dehydroepiandrosterone, 7
Dental care, 31
Depression, puerperal 164
Dermoid cyst, ovary, 287
Desogestrel, 333, 337
Destructive operations, fetal, 185
Diabetes, 104
Diaphragm, contraceptive, 344
Diaphragmatic hernia, fetal, 203
Diarrhoea, infantile, 203
Diazepam, 77
Diet in pregnancy, 31
Diethyl stilhoestrol, 331
Dilatation of cervix, 358
Dilatation and curettage, 358
Discharge, vaginal, 245 et seq.
Disgerminoma, 290
Disproportion, 29, 129
Doderlein's bacilli, 13, 245
Donovan bodies, 240
Down's syndrome, 28
Drugs and the fetus, 113
Ducrey's bacillus, 240
Ductus arteriosus and venosus, 20

Duphaston, 301, 333
Dydrogesterone, 301, 333
Dysfunctional uterine bleeding, 308 et seq.
Dysmenorrhoea, 312 et seq.
Dyspareunia, 319 et seq.
Dystrophia-adiposo-genitalis, 302

Eclampsia, 75
  postpartum, 77
  treatment, 78
Ectopic pregnancy, 69 et seq.
Ectropion, 229, 249
Embedding of fertilized ovum, 16
Embolism, pulmonary 208, 338
  amniotic 153
Embryo, 16 et seq.
Embryotomy, 186
Encephalopathy, 74
Endocrine treatment, 329 et seq.
Endodermal sinus tumour, 288
Endometriosis, 298 et seq.
Endometrium anatomy, 8 et seq.
  atrophic, 251
  biopsy, 322
  carcinoma, 278
  endometritis hyperplasia, 309
  polyp, 269
Endometroid carcinoma of ovary, 287
Engorgement of head, 30, 132
Enterocoele, 233
Entonox, 51
Epidural anaesthesia, 50, 180
Epilepsy, 109
Episiotomy, 51, 125
Epoophoron, 220
Erb's palsy, 202
Ergometrine, 54, 187
Erosion of the cervix, 249
Erythrobastosis fetalis, 168
Essential hypertension, 81
Ethinyl oestradiol, 331
Exchange transfusion, 171
Exenteration, pelvic, 278
External version, 174
  of breech, 124

Extracorporeal fertilization, 327
Eyes, infant, care of, 193

Face presentation, 118
Facial palsy, 201
Fallopian tube, *see* Tube, uterine
Falx cerebri, 42
Feeding, infant, 195 et seq.
Femoral thrombosis, 364
Fenamates, 314
Ferning of cervical mucus, 13, 323
Fertilization, 16
Fetus at risk, 166 et seq.
  asphyxia, 189
  blood sampling, 49
  circulation, 20
  death of, 94
  distress of, 48 et seq.
  drugs affecting, 113
  head measurements, 26, 40
  heart sounds, 23, 30
  injuries, 199 et seq.
  malformations, 26, 128
  maturity, assessment, 94, 186
  measurements, 25, 40
  mortality, 210
  papyraceous, 139
  small for dates, 166
  weight, 39
Fevers, specific, 105
Fibrinous polyp, 270
Fibroma of ovary, 288
Fibromyomata of the uterus, 264 et seq.
Fimbrial cysts, 296
Fistulae, 149
Flagyl, 245
Flushes, 316
Folic acid, 31, 99
Follicle, ovarian, 4
Follicular cyst, 282
Fontanelles, 41
Foramen ovale, 20
Forceps delivery, 175 et seq.
Fothergill operation, 362
Fractures, fetal, 202
Frequency of micturition, 351

INDEX

Frolich's syndrome, 302
FSH, 3, 4, 10, 13
Funic souffle, 23
Funnel pelvis, 130

Gaertner's duct, 219
Galactocoele, 161
Galactorrhoea, 304
Gardnerella vaginalis, 246
Genital ridge, 218
Genital tubercle, 217
Genito-urinary infection, 236 et seq.
Germ cells, 218
Germinal epithelium, 218
Gestadine, 333, 337
Gestogens, see Progestogens
Glycosuria, 103
GnRH, 329
Gonadal agenesis, 220
Gonadotrophic hormones, 3, 5, 8 et seq., 14, 325, 329 et seq.
Gonorrhoea, 107, 236
Graafian follicle, 4
Granuloma inguinale, 240
Granulosa cell tumour, 289
Granulosa cells, 5
Gubernaculum, 218
Guthrie test, 194
Gynaecoid pelvis, 130

Habitual abortion, 66
Haematocoele, pelvic and intraligamentous, 70
Haematocolpos, 222
Haematoma, broad ligament, 70, 149
  vulval, 147
Haemoglobin concentrations
  fetal, 99
  in pregnancy, 98
Haemoglobinopathies, 99
Haemolytic disease, 168 et seq.
Haemophilus Ducreyii, 240
Haemorrhage
  antepartum, 87 et seq.
  infantile, 203
  intracranial, 200
  postpartum, 142 et seq.
Haemorrhagic disease, 203
Haemorrhoids, 112
HCG, 17, 19, 24
Heart disease in pregnancy, 100
Heartburn, 112
Hegar's sign, 23
Hepatic disease, maternal, 109
  of newborn, 204
Hermaphroditism, 226
Heroin addiction, 114
Herpes genitalis, 238
Herpes gestationis, 110
Herpes virus, 107
Hiatus hernia, 112
Hidradenoma, 260
Hirsutes, 304, 307
Hourglass constriction, 137
Hormone releasing intrauterine devices, 342
Hospital booking criteria, 32
Hostile cervical mucus, 327
HPL, 19
Human menopausal gonadotrophin, LMG, 325, 330
Hyaline degeneration of fibroid, 266
Hyaline membrane disease, 192
Hydatidiform mole, 67
Hydrallazine, 77
Hydramnios, 85
Hydrocephaly, 128
Hydrops fetalis, 168
Hydrosalpinx, 252
Hydroxyprogesterone caproate, 333
Hymen, 222
Hyperemesis gravidarum, 74
Hypertension, in pregnancy, 75
Hyperthyroidism, 111
Hypocalcaemia of newborn, 199
Hypofibrinogenaemia, 88
Hypoglycaemia of newborn, 199
Hypotension, supine, 112
Hypotensive drugs, 77 et seq.
Hypothalamus and releasing hormones, 3, 4, 11

Hypothermia of newborn, 193
Hypotonic uterine inertia, 135
Hysterectomy
  abdominal, 364
  vaginal, 362
Hysterosalpingography, 324
Hysteroscopy, 369

Icterus neonatorum, 168
Implants
  contraception, 341
  menopause treatment of, 318
Incarceration of gravid uterus, 234
Incompetence of cervix, 67
Incontinence, urinary, 351
  stress, 352
  urge, 352
Incoordinate uterine action, 135
Induction of labour, 173 et seq.
Induction of ovulation, 325, 326
Infant, birth injuries, 199
  care of newborn, 189 et seq.
  feeding, 195 et seq.
  mortality rate, 210
  small, 197
Infection, prevention of maternal, 46, 57, 154
Infertility, 320 et seq.
Injectable contraception, 340
Injuries, fetal, 199 et seq.
  maternal, 147
Intersex, 225 et seq.
Interstitial salpingitis, 252
Intra-amniotic injection of urea, 349
Intrauterine devices, 341
Intrauterine fetal death, 94
Intrauterine transfusion, 172
Involution of uterus, 56
IVF, 327

Jaundice cholestatic, 338
  maternal, 109
  neonatal, 204

Karman catheter, 348
Kell antigens, 170
Kernicterus, 169
Kidney, see Renal
Kielland's forceps, 176
Kleihauer test, 171
Kleinfelter's syndrome, 225
Kobelt's tubule, 219
Kraurosis, 243
Krukenberg tumour, 290
Kyphoscoliosis, 131

Labia, 222
Labour, normal, 34 et seq.
  augmentation, 47
  delay in, 115
  genital tract abnormalities in, 134
  induction of, 173
  management, 44 et seq.
  mechanism of normal, 42 et seq.
  obstructed, 137
  onset, cause of 34, 43
  premature, 93
  stages, 35 et seq. 49 et seq.
Lactation, 57
  inhibition of, 160
Lactic acid, 245
Lactogen, 19
Laparoscopy, 368
  tubal patency, 324
Laser, 276, 326
Le Fort's operation, 360
Lecithin-sphingomyelin ratio, 187
Leukoplakia vulvae, 243
Levator ani muscle, 44, 231
Levi-loraine syndrome, 302
Levonorgestrel, 333, 337
LH, 3, 4, 13, 17
Libido, female, 7, 10, 15
Lichenification of vulva, 243
Lichensclerosis of vulva, 243
Lie, fetal, 29
Ligaments, pelvic, 230
Linea nigra, 22
Lithopaedion, 71
Liver disease, maternal, 109

INDEX 377

Liver disease (*cont'd*)
  neonatal, 204
Lochia, 56
Locked twins, 140
Lovset's manoeuvre, 125
Lower nephron necrosis, 163
Lower uterine segment, 35
Lupus erythematosus, 82
Lutein cells, 5
Lutein cyst, 283
Lymphogranuloma venerum, 240

Malaria, 106
Malformations, fetal, 26, 128, 129
Malignant disease
  in pregnancy, 111
Manchester operation, 358
Manual removal of placenta, 144
Marshall-Marchetti-
  Krantzoperation, 355
Mastitis, 161
Maternal immune response, 63
Maternal mortality, 208
Maturity, assessment of, 26, 94
McIndoe operation, 222
Meconium, 48
Mefanamic acid, 312
Megaloblastic anaemia, 99
Meig's syndrome, 289
Melanoma of vulva, 261
Membranes, premature rupture, 93
Menarche, 14
Menopause, 14, 15, 316 et seq.
Menstruation
  anovular, 308
  endocrine control, 11 et seq.
  hygiene, 12
  normal cycle, 5, 8 et seq.
Mental disorders, 112
Mental illness in pregnancy, 164
Mento-anterior and posterior
  presentations, 119
Mentum, 41
Mesodermal mixed tumours, 281
Mesonephros, 220
Mesosalpinx, 219

Metastatic carcinoma, 290
Metronidazole, 245
Metropathia haemorrhagica, 309
Milk, composition, 196
Missed abortion, 66
Mole, carneous, 66
  tubal, 72
  vesicular, 67
Moniliasis, 246
Montgomery's tubercules, 22
Morning sickness, 22
Moulding of the head, 40
Mucinous adenocarcinoma, 286
Mucinous cyst adenoma, 283
Mucocolpos, 222
Mullerian ducts, 218
Multiple pregnancy, 138 et seq.
Multiple sclerosis, 110
Muscles, of pelvic floor, 44
  perineal, 38
Mumps, 320
Myasthenia gravis, 110
Myomectomy, 366
Myxoma peritonei, 286

Nabothian follicles, 249
Naegele pelvis, 131
Naloxone, 190
Neonatal mortality, 210
Nephritis, in pregnancy, 82
Nerve injuries, fetal, 201
  maternal, 152
Newborn, *see* Infant
Nipple
  cracked 160
  retracted, 195
Noctural cramps, 113
Norethisterone, 333, 337
Norgestimate, 333, 337
Norgestrel, 333
Nortestosterone, 332

Obstetric statistics, 209 et seq.
Obstructed labour, 137 et seq.
Occipito-posterior and transverse
  position, 116

INDEX

Occiput, 41
Oedema, 76
Oesphageal atresia, 202
Oestrogens, 3, 5, 6, 8 et seq. 17, 330
Oligohydramnios, 86
Oligospermia, 327
Oocyte, 5, 8
Ophthalmia neonatorum, 206
Oral contraception, 335
Ovary
  anatomy, 4, 5
  cysts, 98
  follicle, 3, 4, 5, 11 et seq.
  ovulation, 8
  oxytoxic drugs, 187
  steroids (ovarian), 330
  tumours, 282 et seq.

Pain relief, in labour, 44, 117, 124, 133, 136, 140, 144, 180, 183
Papanicolau stain, 273
Papilliferous carcinoma, ovary, 287
Paralutein cells, 5
Parametritis, 157
Partogram, 47
Pelvic cellulitis, 256
Pelvic haematocoele, 72
Pelvic peritonitis, 256
Pelvis
  abnormalities of, 130
  bones of, 36 et seq.
  cellular tissue, 230
  floor of, 38
  ligaments of, 230
  tumours complicating pregnancy, 95
Pemphigus, 206
Perinatal mortality, 166
Perineal body, 38
  laceration of, 148
Perineal muscles, 231
Perineorrhapy, 360
Peritonitis, puerperal, 157
Pessary, vaginal, 242
Pethidine, in labour, 49
Phaeochromocytoma, 111

Phasic pill (contraception), 337
Phenotype, 223
Phytomenadione (vitamin K1), 204
Piperazine oestradiol sulphate, 317
Pitocin, 187
Pituitary gland, 3
  disorders, 302 et seq.
  hormones, 3, 4, 10, 13, 17
Pituitary necrosis, 163
Pituitary prolactinoma, 111
Placenta, accreta, 143
  abnormalities, 86
  adherent, 143
  anatomy physiology, 3, 17 et seq.
  function tests, 19
  hormones, 17
  insufficiency, 86, 87
  praevia, 90 et seq.
  retained, 146
  separation, 53
Platypelloid pelvis, 130
Polycystic ovary syndrome, 304
Polyhydramnios, 84
Polyneuritis, 74
Polyomyelitis, 106
Polyp, cervical, 270
  placental, 270
Position, fetal, 29
Postcoital test, 323
Posterior pituitary extract, 187
Postmaturity, 94
Postmenopausal bleeding, 316
Postoperative complications, *see under* respective complications
Postnatal examination, 59
Postpartum haemorrhage, 142 et seq.
Precocius puberty, 310
  pre-eclampsia, 75
Pregnancy, 16 et seq.
  abdominal, 70, 721
  antenatal care, 26 et seq.
  breast changes, 22
  diagnosis, 21 et seq. 24
  duration, 21
  ectopic, 69 et seq.

Pregnancy (*cont'd*)
  fibromyomata, and 96, 266
  hypertension in, 75 et seq. 81 et seq.
  intercurrent disease in, 105 et seq.
  laboratory tests for, 24
  multiple, 138 et seq.
  ovarian tumour and, 294
  pelvic tumour and, 95
  prolapse and, 134
  psychological preparation, 31
  retroversion and, 96
  renal transplant in, 84
  symptoms and signs, 21
  vomiting in, 73
Pregnancy induced hypertension, 75
Pregnanediol, 7
Pregnanetriol, 307
Preinvasive cancer, 272 et seq.
Premarin, 331
Premature rupture of membranes, 93
Prematurity, 93, 197
Premenstrual tension, 12, 315
Preparation, for labour, 31
Pre-pregnancy counselling, 27
Presacral nerve and neurectomy, 314
Presentation of cord, 140
Presentation, fetal, 23, 29
Pre-term labour, 93
Primary atrophy of vulva, 242
Procidentia, 232
Progesterone, 3, 6, 8 et seq. 17
Progestogens, 332
  — synthetic
Progestogen only pill, 340
Pronephros, 219
Prostaglandins, 188
Proteinurea, 75 et seq.
Prothrombin deficiency, 203
Pruritus, 110
  vulvae, 244
Prolactin, 4, 304
Prolapse, operations for, 231 et seq.
Prolapse of cord, 140
Prolapse of limbs, 141
Proliferative phase
  menstrual cycle, 8 et seq.
Psychiatric illness, 164
Ptyalism, 74
Puberty, 14
  delayed, 303
Pudental artery, vein and nerve, 39
Pudendal block, 180
Puerperal depression, 164
Puerperal infection, 154 et seq.
Puerperium, 57
  abnormalities of, 154 et seq.
Pulmonary disease in pregnancy, 103
Pulmonary embolism, 162
Purpura, neonatal, 204
Pyelonephritis
  acute, 83
  chronic, 82
Pyosalpinx, 252
Pyrexia, puerperal, 154 et seq.

Quickening, 23

Radiotherapy, for carcinoma of cervix, 276
Radium, 276
Rectocoele, 233
Rectovaginal septum
  endometriosis, 298
Red degeneration of fibroid, 266
Releasing hormones, 3, 308, 329
Renal agenesis
  disease in pregnancy, 82 et seq.
  function in pregnancy, 103
  necrosis, 163
Respiratory distress, 191, 192
Rete ovarii, 220
Retention of urine, 95, 356
Retraction, uterine, 35
  ring, 34
Retroversion of uterus, 235
Reversal of sterilization, 346
Rhesus antibodies, 18, 28

Rhesus antibodies (cont'd)
  factor, 169 et seq.
Rickets, 131
Ring pessary, 234
Ritodrine, 93
Rubella, 105
Rudimetary horn, 221
Rupture of ovarian cyst, 293

Safe period (contraception), 345
Salpingectomy, 367
Salpingography, 324
Salpingolysis, 326
Salpingo-oophoritis, 251 et seq.
Salpingostomy, 326
Sarcoma of uterus, 281
Schiller test, 274
Secretory phase
  menstrual cycle, 8 et seq., 16
Segments, uterine, 35
Seminal fluid, 321
Sepsis, postabortal, 65
  puerperal, 154
Septicaemia, 158
Serous cystadenoma, 286
Sex chromosomes, 223
Sex, determination, 223
  abnormal, 225
Sexual maturation, 13
Sexually transmitted diseases
  in gynaecology, 236 et seq.
  in pregnancy, 107 et seq.
Shared care, in pregnancy, 32
Shirodkar operation, 67
Shock in obstetrics, 153
Shoulders, delivery of
Shoulder presentation, 126
Show, 34
Sickle-cell disease, 99
Simmonds disease, 304
Sinciput, 41
Skin, changes in pregnancy, 22, 110
Skull, fetal, 41
  fractures, 200
Sling operation, 355
Small for dates infants, 197
Smoking and pregnancy, 114

Soft sore, 240
Souffle, 23
Spalding's sign, 95
Sperm antibodies, 323
Sperm penetration test, 323
Spermatozoa, 13, 16
Spermicides, 344
Spinabifida, 128, 186
Spinnbarkeit, 323
Spondylolisthesis, 131
Staphyloccal infection, 155, 161, 205
Stein leventhal syndrome, 304
Sterilisation, 345 et seq.
Stilboestrol, 331
Stillbirth rate, 210
Streptococcal infection, 154, 159, 205
Stress incontinence, 352
Striae gravidarum, 22
Struma ovarii
Succenturiate lobe, 19
Supine hypotension, 112
Surfactant, 189
Symphysiotomy, 185
Syncytiotrophoblast, 17
Syntocinon, 54, 188
Syntometrine, 188
Syphilis, 107, 238

Temperature, basal, 322
Tentorium cerebelli
  tear of, 42
Teratoma, ovary, 287
Termination of pregnancy, 347 et seq.
Testosterone, 333
Testicular feminization, 226
Thalassaemia, 100
Theca interna cells, 5
Theca-lutein cyst, 283
Thecoma, 289
Third stage of labour, 36, 53
Thrombo-cytopenic purpura, 204
Thrombophlebitis, infective, 161
Thrombosis cerebral, 110
  oestrogens and, 338

INDEX

Thrombosis cerebral (*cont'd*)
  postoperative, 357
  venous, 58
Thrush, 246
Thyroid disorders, 305
Torsion of fibromyoma, 266
Torsion of an ovarian tumour, 293
Toxic shock syndrome, 65
Toxoplasmosis, 106
Trachelorrhapy, 229
Transfusion, exchange 171
  intrauterine, 172
Transverse lie, 127
Treponema pallidum, 239
Trial of forceps, 133
Trial of labour, 133
Trichomonitis, 245
Triplets, 138
Trisomy, 186
Trophoblast, 16, 17, 18
Tube, uterine
  development, 218
  ectopic pregnancy, 69
  malformations, 221
  mole, 67
  operations on, 326
  salpingitis, 251
  tests for patency, 324
  tubal abortion, 72
  tumours, 297
Tuberculous endometritis, 248, 251
Tuberculous salpingitis, 257
Tubo-ovarian abscess and cyst, 256
Turner's syndrome, 225
Twins, 138 et seq.

Ultrasonics
  fetal measurement, 25, 30
  pregnancy diagnosis, 25, 26
Umbilical cord
  abnormal insertion, 19
  anatomy, 19
  care of stump, 193
  haemorrhage from, 204
  prolapse of, 140
  vessels of, 18
Ureter, fistula and injury, 352

Urethra, abnormalities of, 262
Urethrovaginal angle, 355
Urinary tract infection, puerperal, 159
Urinary tract, congenital abnormalities, 223
Urinary symptoms, 351 et seq.
Urogenital sinus, 217
Unstable lie, 127
Uterine tube, *see* Tube, uterine
Uterus
  anatomy, 3, 16
  carcinoma, 271 et seq.
  constriction ring, 136
  development, 220
  fibromyomata, 264 et seq.
  incarceration, 95
  incoordinate action, 135 et seq.
  infection, 250
  injury, 228 et seq.
  inversion, 152
  involution, 2
  malformation, 96, 221
  mesodermal missed tumour, 281
  operations on, 364
  polyp, 270
  retraction, 35
  retroversion, 235
  rupture, 47, 149, 229
  sarcoma, 281
  segments, 35
  souffle, 23
  supports of, 230
  see also Cervix and Endometrium

Vaccination, 106
Vacuum extraction, 179
Vagina anatomy, 218
  atresia, 222
  atrophic changes, 247
  congenital abnormalities, 221
  development, 218
  diaghragm, contraceptive, 334
  discharge from, 245
  examination, 451
  injections, 245 et seq.
  inversion, 235

Vagina anatomy (*cont'd*)
  injury of fistulae, 228
  lacerations, 149, 228
  prolapse, 231
  secretion, 245
  support of, 230
  tumours, 263
  vaginitis, 245
Vaginal rings (contraception), 341
Vaginismus, 319
Varicocoele, 320
Varicose veins, 112
Vasa previa, 19
Vasectomy, 347
Velamentous insertion of cord, 19
Venereal disease, 236
Venous thrombosis, puerperal, 161
Ventouse, 179
Ventrosuspension, 234
Vernix caseosa, 193
Vesicovaginal fistulae, 228, 351, 352
Vesicular mole, 67
Version, 174
Vitamin K, 204
Vomiting in pregnancy, 73
  of newborn, 202
Vulvitis, 241 et seq.
Vulva,
  anatomy, 217
  atrophic change, 243
  condylomata, 242
  dysplasia, 243
  excision, 244
  haematoma, 147
  injury, 147
  kraurosis, 243
  leukoplakia, 243
  lichen sclerosis, 243
  operations on, 359
  pruritis, 244
  tumours, 260
  varix, 113
  vulvitis, 241
  warts, 242

Warfarin, 162, 364
Wertheim's hysterectomy, 97, 278
Wharton's jelly, 19
William's operation, 223
Wolffian ducts, 218
Wrigley' forceps, 175

XY chromosomes, 223

Yolk sac, 218

Zygote, 16